an illustrated
guide to
medical
terminology

an illustrated guide to medical terminology

HELEN R. STRAND

The Williams & Wilkins Co.

BALTIMORE · 1968

FOREWORD

The author of this book came to my office in November 1962 and has remained with me ever since as Chief Personal and Confidential Secretary. In my position at that time as Chairman of the Department of Surgery, she was immediately thrown into a vortex of many and varied duties as is usual in a Department with almost 200 staff members, a complicated budget and many personalities with which to deal. All this she handled in masterful fashion. Soon I began to hear about the "book" which she was preparing in off-duty time. At first I was skeptical, but then as I was shown the general format and later some of the chapters I became first convinced and later enthusiastic. For over two years my advice regarding this project has been sought and willingly given.

There are three features of prime importance regarding Miss Strand's monograph which seem of especial significance to me. *First*, there is a need for such a book. With the ever expanding scope of medical schools, hospitals, research laboratories and drug firms, the supply of good medical secretaries falls far short of the demand. Whereas training of business secretaries is a highly developed art, the training of medical secretaries is largely a hit-or-miss affair. No book of which I am aware supplies this need as well as does that by Miss Strand. In succinct fashion it outlines and correlates the terminology which a medical secretary should know with both basic word roots and with basic medical knowledge. Without these correlations, the secretary's use of the terminology would be mere rote and hence far less useful.

Second, as an experienced and competent medical secretary, Miss Strand knows whereof she writes.

Third, to me the book seems well planned and clearly written. I am pleased to endorse it. I would even go so far as to state that the reading of it might not only benefit all medical secretaries, medical librarians, drug salesmen, hospital administrative officers and other lay persons who constantly must deal with medical terminology, but it might benefit some medical students and doctors as well.

Henry N. Harkins, M.D., Ph.D., F.A.C.S.*
Professor of Surgery
University of Washington School of Medicine
Seattle, Washington 98105

*Deceased 12 August 1967.

PREFACE

The instigating factor in writing this book was a course which the author once took on medical terminology which demonstrated the need for a simple, clear and concise presentation of the subject particularly for medical secretaries, but also for all others who utilize medical terms.

The two special features of the book are to give the "key" to medical terminology in general and then to particularize it as "medical terminology at a glance" utilizing illustrations of the different body systems. These two features are presented in that order, since it seemed logical to first learn the basis or key to medical terminology and then to progress into the mechanics of language pertaining to the different systems of the body.

The graphic approach is utilized to a considerable degree in clarifying the second feature of the book. It is difficult to separate medical terminology itself from the subject matter which it describes. Consequently, a condensation of anatomy and some physiology is included in the respective introductory chapters to each of the 11 body systems. Medical terminology is illustrated relating to each separate system, followed in each instance by an outline of the surgical procedures relating to the respective systems. Finally, there are concluding chapters on "Diseases," "Anesthesiology," "Radiology," and "Pathology."

The author would like to take this opportunity to thank the many personal friends who were encouraging in the development of this work, and the co-workers here at the University of Washington who so patiently listened to the plans outlined for it, and particularly to Dr. Henry N. Harkins who really gave the first professional encouragement as to whether it should be written at all!

Special thanks are extended to Dr. Robert F. Mullarky for time spent in checking the first draft of the manuscript; to Dr. L. Stanton Stavney for his thorough review of the completed manuscript; to Dr. Loren Winterscheid for his advice and guidance in writing the Cardiovascular Chapter; to Dr. Alfred A. Strauss for his review of the completed manuscript; to Drs. Lawrence M. Knopp and James R. S. Paterson and to Dr. Henry N. Harkins for his final word on the manuscript.

The author is indebted to the following for illustrations: from *Stedman's Medical Dictionary, 21st ed.*, Basmajian: *Primary Anatomy, 5th ed.* and Grant & Basmajian: *Grant's Method of Anatomy, 7th ed.*; from Dorland's Medical Dictionary, published by W. B. Saunders Company; to Miss Jessie Phillips, Mrs. Marjorie Domenowske and Mrs. Phyllis Wood in the Medical Illustration Department of the University of Washington for their work; to the Medical Photography Department of the University of Washington for their fine work; and to Dr. Jack Rudick for his assistance in some of the photography work.

Now, some three years later the end result is presented. It is hoped that all those who use medical terminology, particularly medical secretaries, will find it interesting and helpful.

Helen R. Strand
Department of Surgery
University of Washington School of Medicine
Seattle, Washington

CONTENTS

I

THE KEY TO MEDICAL TERMINOLOGY

ROOTS

There is no point where art so nearly touches nature as when it appears in the form of words. HOLLAND, PLAIN TALKS ON FAMILIAR SUBJECTS. ART AND LIFE.

Root words are the key to a working knowledge of Greek and Latin vocabulary so pertinent to acquiring a medical vocabulary. Root terms which form the basis for some 4000 medical words are listed alphabetically, e.g., *aden* relating to gland or *bio* relating to life. From these roots, primarily of Greek and Latin origin, medical terminology receives its derivation, the root word occurring frequently in its various forms.

A root is an element common to all the words of a group of similar meaning, remaining after the formative additions, prefixes or suffixes, have been removed.

Everyday terms that appeared in ancient medical Latin include: abdomen, anus, cancer, delirium, tibia, valgus and varus (Celsus, *fl.* 30 A.D.); and acetabulum, tinea and verruca (Pliny, 23–79 A.D.). However, other language sources have given us the following terminology.

From Arabic, we derive our pharmacopeia, e.g., alcohol, alkali, camphor, naphtha, senna, syrup and tartar. Prefixing the Arabic article *al* and *el* to a Greek stem, e.g., *al*-chemy, *el*-ixir, we form others.

From Anglo-Saxon, come our most simple anatomical terms: arm, back, bladder, blood, chin, eye, finger, foot, gall, gum, gut, hair, hand, head, heart, hip, knee, liver, lung, mouth, neck, thumb and tongue, as well as ache, fat, hives, sick and swell. A few words of Scandinavian descent are ill, leg, scab and skin.

Medical terms adopted from the French and unchanged or slightly modified are: ballottement, bougie, chancre, cretin, curette, fontanelle, fourchette, grippe, malaise, pipette, plaque, poison, rale, souffle, tampon, tourniquet, trocar, venom, cul de sac, grand mal, petit mal, mal der mer and tic douloureux. Some Anglicized or Americanized forms of French words are goiter, gout, malady, malinger, jaundice, ointment, physician and powder, while still others come from the Greek through a French intermediary, e.g., surgeon, plaster, migraine, quinsy, palsy and frenzy.

From Italian, we have a few words such as belladonna, influenza, and malaria.

We are indebted to Spanish for certain terms relating to medicaments, *e.g.*, cascara, and quaiacum; and to the Dutch for cough, litmus, splint and sprue; to German for anlage, Fahrenheit and magenstrasse; to Persian for bezoar, borax and talc.

Most of our present vocabulary has been in use for 2000 years or more. Hippocrates (460–370 B.C.) used the following words: acromion, adenoma, amblyopia, anthrax, apophysis, borborygumus, bregma, bronchus, cachexia, carcinoma, cholera, erythema, exanthema, herpes, hippus, ileus, kyphosis, lichen, lochia, lordosis, meninges, nephritis, noma, nystagmus, olecranon, paresis, peritoneum, phagedena, phthisis, polypus, psilosis, symphysis, thorax, typhus, urachus, ureter and urethra. Galen (131–201 A.D.) included in his medical vocabulary such words as anthrax, aponeurosis, ascites, chalazion, chemosis, coccyx, diaphoresis, diastole, epididymis, epiphora, gomphosis, hippus, hypophysis, hypospadias, iris, kerion, lysis, mydriasis, pemphigus, peritoneum, phimosis, pityriasis, pterygium, pylorus, sacroma, skeleton, strabismus, syndrome, systole, tarsus, tenia, thymus, tinea and trichiasis. Aristotle (384–322 B.C.) made use of the following terms: alopecia, canthus, exophthalmos, glaucoma, leukoma, meconium, nystagmus, pancreas and podagra.

A large group of words comprise those formed from nonmedical origins, *e.g.*, anthrax, a hot coal; pancreas, all-flesh; pylorus, gatekeeper; scaphoid, boatlike; trochlear (trochlea), pulley.

Even living creatures have loaned their descriptive names to medical terminology: cancer (L. crab), carcinoma (G. *karkinos*, crab); hippocampus (seahorse), cauda equina (horse's tail), lumbrical (L. *lumbricus*, worm), vermis (L. worm), cochlea (G. snail), chemosis (G. *cheme*, cockle-shell), lupus (L. wolf), muscle (L. *musculus*, little mouse), buphthalmos (G. ox-eyed), lagophtalmos (hare-eyed), ichthyosis (G. *ichthus*, fish), phrynoderma (G. toadskin), estrus (G. *oistros*, gadfly), formication (L. *formica*, ant), coccyx (G. cuckoo), coronoid (G. *korone*, crow), coracoid (G. *korax*, crow), chenopodium (G. *chene*, goose), rostrum (L. beak). Wings from both Latin (ala, axilla, pinna) and Greek (pterion, pterygium, pterygoid). The horse's accouterment is represented by stapes (stirrup) and sella (saddle).

Weapons and arms are also freely used: the club (coryne-), sword (xiphoid, ensiform), sheath (vagina), bow (toxic), arrow (sagittal), helmet (galea), shield (thyroid, umbo, umbilicus) and breastplate (thorax). Musical instruments are also represented: salpinx (G. trumpet), tympanum, (L. drum), calamus, (L. reed), fistula, (L. pipe)

and syrinx (G. pipe); and only one musician is mentioned, the trumpeter (buccinator).

Utensils and household items also contributed to medical terminology: *Pyelos*, a pan or basin, gives us pyelitis, inflammation of the kidney pelvis (platypelloid); *amnion* and *pellis* are Greek words for bowls; patella (L.) is a small pan, platysma is a flat plate (G.); arytenoid from *arytania* (G.) is a ladle; ascites comes from *askos* (G.), a leather wineskin, and acetabulum (L.), a little saucer for vinegar. The ampulla was a jar (L.). Calyx and cotyle (*cotyloid, cotyledon*) were Grecian drinking cups; sieves have given us cribriform and ethymoid; and finally infundibulum is a funnel (L.).

The grapevine plays a major role in its contribution to our medical terminology. *Uva* is Latin for the grape itself and gives us uvea and uvula. *Botrys* and *staphyle* are two Greek words meaning a bunch of grapes, and *racemus* is their Latin equivalent; hence, our words staphylococcus, botryoid and racemose. All of these describe objects which give the appearance of clustering grapes or berries. The vine itself gives us our pampiniform plexus (*pampinus*, tendril).

Then we have acquired words related to fruits. These include pyriform (pear-shaped), sycosis (G. *sykon*, a fig), morula (L. *morum*, a blackberry), nucleus, a little nut (L. *nux*, nut), karyo- (G. *karyon*, nut), glans (L. acorn) and balanitis (G. *balanos*, acorn), myrtiformes (shaped like myrtle berries), pomum Adami (Adam's apple), streptococcus and other cocci (G. *kokkos*, berry).

Finally, vegetables and other crops, such as grains, are also represented in the formation of our medical terminology such as pisiform (pea-shaped), hordeolum (L. *hordeum*, barley), pityriasis (G. *pityra*, bran), sesamoid (G. *sesamon*, sesame seed), aphakia (G. *phakos*, lentil), lens (L. *lentil*), and fabella (a little bean).

Following is an alphabetical list of roots with their meanings.

AC- Sharpness.	ADIP- Fat.	AMBLY- Blunt, dull.
ACOU- To hear.	AER- Air.	AMEB-, AMOEB- Change,
ACT, AG- To lead, drive.	ALB- White.	alteration.
ACTIN- A ray, beam.	ALG- Pain.	AMNI- A bowl, membrane.
ADEN- A gland.	ALI-, ALL- Other, another.	AMYL-, see MYL-

ANC-, ANG-, ANK- A bend or hollow.

ANDR- A man.

ANGI- A vessel, usually blood vessel.

ANTH- A flower.

ANTHR- Charcoal.

ANTR- A cave, cavity of body.

AORT- Original.

AQU- Water.

ARACH- A spider; spider's web.

ARCH- Beginning, origin.

ARG- Shining, bright

ARTER- The windpipe; an artery as distinct from a vein.

ARTH- A joint; a connecting word.

ARTIC- A joint.

ASTER-, ASTRO- A star.

ASTH- A short drawn breath.

ASTRAG- A vertebra; ball of the ankle joint.

ATM- Steam, vapor.

AUD-, AUR-, AUS- To hear.

AUX- Increase in power; strengthen.

BAC- A rod-shaped structure; microorganism.

BACT- A staff; unicellular microörganism.

BALAN- An acorn; pessary, a suppository.

BALL-, BEL-, BOL- To throw

BAS-, BET- A step, base.

BIO- Life.

BLAST- A sprout, shoot; of animals, the germ.

BLEN- A thick mucous discharge.

BLEP- To see.

BRACHI- Arm.

BRACHY- Short.

BRANCH- A fin.

BRONCH- The trachea, the windpipe.

BUB- The groin; a swelling in the groin.

BUCC- The cheek (area around the mouth).

BURS- A purse; in anatomy, a pouch or sac.

CAD-, CID- To fall.

CALL- Hard, thick skin; insensibility.

CALX-, CALCA- The heel.

CALX-, CALCI-, CALCO- Limestone, lime.

CAMP- To bend.; flexible.

CANC- A crab; a malignant tumor.

CAP-, CEP-, CIP- The head.

CAP-, CEPT-, CIP- To seize, take.

CARB- Coal, charcoal.

CARC- A crab; ulcer, cancer.

CARD-, CARDI- Heart; mind; the cardiac extremity of the stomach.

CAROT- The great arteries of the neck; to plunge into heavy sleep.

CARP- The joint of the hand and the arm; the wrist.

CARP- A simple pistil.

CAUS-, CAUT- To set on fire, burn; of surgeons, to cauterize.

CELE- A tumor, a rupture.

CELI-, COELI-, CELO- Hollow, or any cavity.

CELL- A storeroom, a chamber. A cell, a miniature structure.

CENT-, CEST- Prick, stab; a puncture of a cavity.

CEPHAL- Head.

CERAS-, CRAS- Mix, or mingle.

CERAT-, KERAT- The horn of an animal; a horny structure.

CES-, CAES-, CID-, CIS- To strike, cut.

CHEIL- Lip.

CHEM- Transmuting the baser metals into gold.

CHIR-, CHEIR- The hand.

CHLOR- Green.

CHOL- Gall, bile.

CHOND- Groats of wheat; gristle, or cartilage.

CHORD-, CORD- Guts, a string of the guts.

CHORI- The membrane that encloses the fetus.

CHROM-, CHROS- The surface of the body; a complexion, color.

CHY- To pour.

CIL- Eyelash; a hairlike process.

CIN-, KIN- To set in motion; sense of movement.

CION- The uvula; a pillar or column.

CLAS- To break; or deflected (of lines or rays).

CLAUS-, CLUS-, CLUD- Close, shut.

CLEID-, CLEIS-, CLID- To close, bar, enclose.

CLIM-, CLIN-, CLIV- To make bend, or recline.

COCC- A grain, seed.

COCCY- A cuckoo; the os coccygis (resemblance of a cuckoo's bill).

COCH- A snail; a spiral.

COLL- A glue, a derivative of gelatin.

COLL- The neck; any necklike part.

COLP- Vagina.

COND- A knuckle, of any joint.

COPR- Feces.

CORD- A maiden, a puppet; the pupil of the eye (because a little image appears in it).

CORI- Hide, skin.

CORN- A horn; anything of horny substance.

CORON- A kind of crow; shaped or hooked like the bill of a crow.

CORP- Any body or mass; the main part of an organ.

COST- Rib.

CRANI- Skull.

CRES-, CRET- To grow, arise, increase.

CRET-, CREM- To separate; to distinguish.

CRI- To separate, distinguish; bring to a crisis.

CRY- Icy cold.

CUB- To recline, lie down (thus, the elbow, on which one reclines).

CUSS-, CUT- To shake, agitate.

CY-, CYT- To conceive, be pregnant.

CYAN- A dark blue substance.

CYC- A ring, circle, or any circular body.

CYN- A dog; unilateral facial paralysis.

CYST- The bladder.

DER- The skin, the outer tegument.

DES- To bind, tie.

DEUT- Second.

DIDY- Twofold, twin.

DIG- A finger or toe; usually a finger, as distinguished from dactylous, a toe.

DIPH- A prepared hide, leather.

DOCH-, DOC- Take, receive; a holder, receptacle.

DREP- A sickle.

DROM- A running, a race.

DUC-, DUCT- To lead, guide.

EC-, OEC- A house, chamber.

ECHIN- A hedgehog; a sea-urchin. Having the sense of roughness.

ECHO- A sound. A reverberating sound.

ECT-, EX-, HEX-, SCH-, OCH- To have, hold.

EDEM-, OEDEM- A swelling, a tumor.

ELECT- Amber. (The process of developing electricity was first observed in amber.)

ELYT- A cover; the sheath.

EMB- A young animal. A fetus.

ENCEPHAL- Brain.

ENTER- A piece of gut; the intestines.

ER- To take, grasp.

ERG-, ORG- Work; the unit of work, or in the metric system.

ERYTH- Red.

ES-, ET-, HET- To let go, release.

ESOPH- see PHAG-

EST-, AESTH- Perception by the senses.

ETH-, AETH- The sky, heaven.

ETI-, AETI- A charge, the cause.

FAC-, FEC-, FIC-, To make, build.

FACI- Form, shape, face.

FEC-, FAEC- Grounds, dregs, refuse - feces.

FER-, FERT- To bear.

FIS-, FID- To cleave, split.

FLAG- A whip; a young branch.

FLAT- To blow, inflate.

FLECT-, FLEX- To bend.

FLU-, FLUX- To flow.

FOLL- A small bag; shell.

FOR- To bore, pierce.

FORN- An arch or vault, a structure of the brain.

FRA- To break into pieces.

FUN-, FUS- To pour; melt, diffuse.

GAL-, GALACT- Milk.

GAM- Being. A sexual form.

GANGL- A tumor under the skin.

GANGR- An eating sore.

GASTER-, GAST- The stomach.

GEN-, GON- The sense of become, beget, produce.

GEST- To bear, carry, to produce.

GLAN- An acorn. A gland.

GLI- Glue. A gluelike mass.

GLO- A round body, a ball.

GNO- To discern, know; knowledge.

GON-, GONY- The knee.

GRAM-, GRAPH- To scratch; write.

GYN- A woman.

HAB-, HIB- To have, to hold. Condition or state of a thing.

HAEM-, HEM-, -EM Blood.

HAP-, AP- To fasten to. A binding together.

HELIC- Any spiral shape, the convolution of a shell.

HELM- An intestinal worm.

HEPAT- The liver.

HERM- Airtight, hermetic. Hermes, the god of the arts and sciences.

HERN- A rupture, hernia.

HETER- Other; different.

HIPP- A horse. In medicine, a complaint of the eyes such that they are always winking.

HIST- Anything set upright; in anatomy, tissue; histoblast.

HOD-, -OD A way, path; method.

HOM-, -OM- One and the same.

HUM- The upper arm.

HYDR- Water.

HYGR- Fluid, moist.

HYL-, -YL Matter, material and pulp tissues.

HYST- The womb; the ovary of animals.

HYST- Later, following.

ICHOR- The ethereal juice that flows in the veins of the gods instead of blood; a discharge, the thin watery discharge from an ulcer.

ICHTH- A fish.

IDIO- One's own.

INGUI- The front part of the body between the hips and the groin.

INI-, INO- Muscle; (later) the fibrous vessels in the muscles.

INSUL- An island. Any circumscribed body.

IRIS, IRID- Any bright colored circle, the iris of the eye.

ISCH- To hold back; suppression of any discharge.

ISCHI- The hip joint.

-ITIS Inflammation of.

JAC-, JEC- Throw, hurl. To utter.

JEJ- Fasting, hungry. Jejunum, so called because it is supposed to be empty after death.

JUNC-, JUG- To join together.

LAB-, LEPS-, LEPT- To take hold of, receive.

LABYR- A maze. A labyrinth, the internal ear.

LACT- Milk.

LAL- Talk, chatter.

LARV- A ghost, specter, a mask. The wormlike form of an insect.

LEC- The yolk of an egg.

LEN- A lens, because of its shape like that of a split lentil.

LEP- To strip.

LEUK White.

LEV- Left.

LIG- To tie; bandage.

LING-, LIG- Pertaining to the tongue.

LITH- A stone.

LOG- A word, speech, discourse.

LOPH- The back of the neck. Tufted.

LY-, LYS- To loosen, unfasten. Dissolve.

LYMPH- Water, a clear fluid.

MAG-, MANG- A magnet; a silverlike mineral.

MAL-, MALI- Bad. Malnutrition; malignant.

MALAC-, MALAG- Soft, gentle. Softening of tissues.

MANI- Madness.

MANI-, MANU- Hand.

MARA-, MARC- A wasting away; decay.

MAT-, METR- The womb.

MEA- To go, pass. An external opening.

MED- Middle.

MEG- Great.

MEL- Honey.

MEL- Fruit.

MEL- A limb.

MEL- A song.

MELAN-, MELEN- Black.

MEN-, MENS- A month, refers to the menses.

MENIN- Any membrane, primarily that of the brain.

MER- Part.

MIO-, MEIO- Lesser.

MIST-, MIX- To mix, mingle.

MNEM-, MNES- To remind, memory.

MOLAR- A mill, A jawbone.

MOLEC-, MOLI- A shapeless, heavy mass.

MOLL- Soft, delicate.

MORB- Grief, distress.

MORPH- Form, or shape.

MOV-, MOT-, MOB- Set in motion.

MUSC- A fly.

MUSCU-, MUSCL-, MY- A mouse; a muscle of the body.

MYC- A mushroom.

MYEL- Marrow.

MYI- A fly.

MYL- A mill, grinders.

MYO- To close the eyes.

NAPH- A clear, combustible rock oil.

NEB-, NEPH- Mist, vapor; fog, or cloudlike.

NERV-, NEUR- Sinew, nerve.

NEST- Fasting.

NITR- Nitrate.

NOCT-, NYCT- Night.

NOM- Custom, usage.

NOMEN-, NOMIN- A name.

NUC-, NUX A nut.

NYMPH- A bride; a married woman.

OCN-1 Bulk, mass of a body.

OCN-2 A hook, any angle.

OCUL- The eye, or resemblance thereto.

-OD, see HOD.

ODYN- Pain of body or mind.

-OID, -ODE Form, shape.

OMEN- Adipose membrane. Fat. Any skin that encloses an internal part of the body.

ONT- To be, present part of, as the history of the evolution of an individual.

OO- An egg.

ODONT- Tooth.

OMO- Shoulder.

OOPHOR- Ovary.

OPH- The eye.

OPIO-, OPO- Animal extracts.

OPO-, OPS-, OMM- To see; sight.

OPSI- Late.

OPSO- Cooked meat; a seasoning. In medicine, an element found in serum.

ORCH- A testicle.

ORO- The watery part of blood, serum.

ORTH- Straight; upright.

OS-, OR- The mouth.

OS, OSS-, OST- A bone.

OSM-, OZ-, -OD- Older form; a smell, odor. Sense of smell.

OT- An ear.

OV- An egg; egg-shaped.

OVIN- Relating to a sheep.

OX- Sharp. Keen.

PAG-, PECT-, PEX- To make fast; as of liquids, to freeze.

PALM- PALMO- A quivering motion; pulsation.

PALP- To touch softly.

PAN- All, every; the whole.

PARI-, PART- To bring forth, bear, to produce.

PARIE- A wall, as of the chest.

PAT- To lie open.

PATH- Disease.

PED-, PAED- A Child.

PELV-, PELY- The pelvis, any basin or cup-shaped cavity.

PENI- The penis.

PEP- To cook, to digest.

PES-, PED- The foot; or a footlike part of anything.

PHAG- To eat.

PHAN-, PHEN-, PHAS- Bring to light; show.

PHEM-, PHAS- A voice.

PHER-, PHOR- To bear, carry.

PHIL- To love.

PHLEG-, PHLOG- To burn; to flame; inflammation.

PHO- Light.

PHRAG-, PHRAX- To fence in. Hedgeround.

PHTH- To decline, waste away.

PHYLL- A leaf; arrangement of leaves on a stem.

PHYS- A pair of bellows; a breath.

PITU- Secreting or containing mucus.

PLAC- A cake; the organ of attachment of the fetus to the wall of the uterus.

PLAS- To form, mold.

PLES-, PLEX-, PLEG- To strike.

PLEUR- A rib, the side; the serous membrane which envelops the lung.

PLIC-, PLEX- To fold, wind together.

PN-, PNEU- To blow; breathe. Relating to the lungs.

POD- A foot.

POLIO- Gray.

POR- A river ford; a passage through, such as the pore of the skin.

POR- A kind of marble; a node on the bones; stone in the bladder.

PORPH-, PURP- The purple fish; the dye obtained from it; purple.

PRAG-, PRAC-, PRAX- To do; the science of conduct.

PRISM- Something sawn; a geometric prism.

PROCT- Anus.

PSEUD- To deceive. False.

PSYCH- The mind.

PTER- A wing.

PTOM-, PTOS- A fall; a corpse.

PTY- To spit out.

PUNC- To prick, puncture.

PUP- A girl; a doll. A stage in the development of an insect.

PUR-, PUS- Pus.

PYEL- A tub; vat. In compounds, the pelvis.

PYR- Fire; violent fever.

PYTH-, PYO- To decay.

QUAD-, QUAR- Four.

QUANT- Amount.

QUERC- The bark of; an oak tree.

RAB- Rage, madness.

RADI- A staff; spoke of a wheel.

REG-, RECT-, RIG- To keep straight; guide.

RET- A net.

RHACH-, RACH- The spine, the backbone.

RHAG-, RHEG-, RHEX-, -RRHAG To break; shatter. Burst.

RHAPH-, -RRHEA-, RHY- To sew; suture.

RHE-, -RRHE- To flow.

RHIN- The nose.

RUB- Red.

RUPT- To break, burst.

SACC- A sac, bag.

SACCH- Sugar.

SALP- A trumpet; in anatomy, a tube.

SANG-, SANI- Blood.

SAPR- Rot.

SARC- Flesh; a bud from a germinating cell.

SCHI-, SCISS- To split, separate.

SCLER- Hard.

SCOP- To look at, behold.

SEB-, SEV- A concretion in a sebaceous follicle.

SEC-, SEG- To cut.

SEP-, SEPS-, SEPT- To make rotten, poison.

SEPT- Seven.

SER- The watery part of things, such as blood after coagulation.

SINU- A curve; a hollow.

SIT- Food.

SKEL- Dried up.

SOLU-, SOLV- Release, dissolve.

SOM- The body as opposed to the spirit.

SPA- To draw, stretch; in medicine, to cause spasm.

SPER-, SPOR- To sow, seed.

SPHIN- A band, such as a muscle closing an aperture.

SPHYG-, SPHYX- To throb; to beat.

SPIR- A coil.

SPIR- To breathe.

SPLAN- The inward parts, such as internal organs.

SPLEN- The ancients believed to be the seat of anger and melancholy. Relating to the spleen.

STA-, STEM- Stand, or set up.

STAL-, STOL- Set, or place; a restriction.

STAPH- Relating to grapes.

STERN- The chest.

STHEN- Strength.

STIG- Mark of a pointed instrument. A mark, spot.

STOM- The mouth, or any outlet or entrance.

STREP-, STRO- To turn; twist.

STYP- Draw together, contract.

SUD- Sweat.

SULC- A furrow, grooves, depression.

SULF-, SULPH- Brimstone, sulphur.

SYRI- A pipe, or tube.

TACH- Swift.

TACT-, TAG-, TIG- To touch, tangible.

TAL- The ankle, heel.

TAR- A broad flat surface.

TAX-, TACT- To arrange.

TEMP- Time, the right place.

TEN-, TON-, TAS- To stretch, strain.

TEST- A shell, a seed covering.

TEST- A testicle.

THE- Set, place.

THEL- The nipple.
THER- To tend.
THYM- Thyme.
THYM- The soul, mind.
THYR- A door.
TOM- To cut.
TONS- The tonsils.
TORS-, TORT- To turn, twist, a wringing.
TOX- A bow. Arrow poison.
TRACH- Rough.
TRACH- The neck, throat.
TREM-, TRES- To bore through; perforation.
TREP-, TROP- To turn.
TREPH- To increase, support, rear.

TRIB-, TRIP-, TRYP-, TREP- To rub, bruise, crush.
TRICH- The hair.
TYP- A blow; mark of a blow; impression.
TYPH- Smoke; stupor arising from fever.
TYPHL- Blind.
UL- A scar.
UL- The gums.
UR- Urine.
UV- A grape, or shaped like a grape.
VACC- Relating to a cow.
VAGI- The covering sheath.
'VARI- A dilated vein. Bent, stretched.

VARI- Diverse. Different.
VECT-, VET-, VEX- To bear, to carry.
VEL- A curtain, or resembling a veil.
VENT- Anything that swells, or bellies out.
VERT-, VORT- To turn, change position.
VISC-' A glutinous substance from mistletoe; clammy, sticky.
XEN- Guest; host; foreigner.
XER- Dry.
ZE-, ZY- To boil.
ZO- To live.

GREEK AND LATIN LETTER COMBINATIONS

In the Greek language we have the following combinations of letters which are peculiar to Greek spelling:

A few of the more common singular and plural endings peculiar to Greek and Latin are:*

Combination	Word	Singular	Plural
ch for k	Chyle	A. . .Macula	Ae. . .Maculae
cn for n	Cnemitis	Ex. . .Index	Ces. . .Indices
gn for n	Gnosia	Is. . .Psychosis	Es. . .Psychoses
ph for f	Physiology	On. . .Phenomenon	A. . .Phenomena
pn for n	Pneumonia	Um. . .Antrum	A. . .Antra
ps for s	Psittacosis	Us. . .Bacillus	I. . .Bacilli
rh for r	Rhinitis	Itis. . .Arthritis	Itides. . .Arthritides

ENGLISH, GREEK AND LATIN SINGULARS AND PLURALS MOST FREQUENTLY USED IN MEDICAL WRITING

Singular	Plural	Singular	Plural
addendum	addenda	appendix	appendices
adenoma	adenomata	aqua	aque
ala	ala	arcus	arcus
albacans	albacantes	areola	areolae
alveolar	alveoli	ascaris	ascarides
amygdala	amygdalae	ascus	asci
antenna	antennae	atrium	atria
antiad	antiades	axilla	axillae
antrum	antra	axis	axes
apertura	aperturae	bacterium	bacteria
aperture	apertures	bronchus	bronchi
apex	apices	bulla	bullae
aponeurosis	aponeuroses	bursa	bursae

*From Smither, Effie: Gregg Medical Shorthand Manual, 2nd Ed. McGraw-Hill Book Co., Inc. N.Y. 1949

Singular	Plural	Singular	Plural
cactus	cacti	foramen	foramina
cadaver	cadavera	formula	formulas, formulae
calcaneum	calcanea	fossa	fossae
cantharis	cantharides		
canthus	canthi	ganglion	ganglia
cannula	cannulas	gland	glands
carcinoma	carcinomas	glaucoma	glaucomas
chondroma	chondromas	gonad	gonads
commissura	commissurae	gonococcus	gonococci
condyloma	condylomas	gum	gumas
conjunctiva	conjunctivae	gyrus	gyri
cornea	corneas		
cornu	cornua	hematoma	hematomas
corpus	corpora	index	indices
cortex	cortices	ilium	ilia
crisis	crises	keratosis	keratoses
criterion	criteria	labium	labia
cuniculus	cuniculi	lamella	lamellae
curriculum	curriculums, curricula	lamina	laminae
		lipoma	lipomas
datum	data	loculus	loculi
deferens	deferentia	locus	loci
dens	dentes		
diagnosis	diagnoses	maxilla	maxillae
diaphoreticus	diaphoretici	medium	media
diastema	diastemata	micra, micron	micras, microns
digitus	digiti	mucosa	mucosae
diverticulum	diverticula	myoma	myomas
dorsum	dorsi	myxoma	myxomas
echolatus	echolati	nevus	nevi
embolus	emboli	naevus	naevi
endothelioma	endotheliomas	nodulus	noduli
enema	enemas, enemata	nodus	nodi
ensis	enses	noxa	noxae
epididymis	epididymides	nucleus	nuclei
epithelioma	epitheliomas		
erythema	erythemas	ovum	ova
esthesis	estheses	os	ora
exanthem	exanthemata		
		papilla	papillae
fascia	fasciae	pathema	pathemata
fasciculus	fasciculi	perineum	perinea
fibroma	fibromata	pernio	perniones
filix	filices	petechia	petechiae
filum	fila	pilus	pili
fistula	fistulas, fistulae	pilula	pilulae
flagellum	flagella	plasma	plasmas
focus	foci	pleura	pleurae
folliculus	folliculi	polypus	polypi
fomis	fomites	protozoon	protozoa

Singular	Plural	Singular	Plural
psammoma	psammomas	sudamen	sudamina
		sulcus	sulci
quadruplet	quadruplus		
quotient	quotient	tarsus	tarsi
		tela	telae
radius	radii	tinctura	tincturae
ramus	rami	toxicosis	toxicoses
		trauma	traumas, traumata
sanitarium	sanitariums	typha	typhae
sanitorium	sanitoriums		
sarcoma	sarcomas	ulcus	ulcera
scotomas	scotomata	uterus	uteri
septum	septa		
sequela	sequelae		
sequestrum	sequestra	varix	varices
serosa	serosae	vas	vasa
spasmus	spasmi	verruca	verrucae
spectrum	spectra	vertebra	vertebrae
speculum	specula	vesical	vesicals
sperma	spermata	vesicula	vesiculae
spermatozoon	spermatozoa	vis	vires
sputum	sputa	viscus	viscera
stimulus	stimuli	vomica	vomicae
stigma	stigmata		
stoma	stomata	zygoma	zygomata

PREFIXES

With the knowledge of the meaning of the foregoing medical terms—prefixes, suffixes and combining forms (both prefixes and suffixes)—it is comparatively easy to dissect many medical words so that their meaning is automatically revealed. Several examples are as follows. Pericarditis: *peri* (around), *card* (heart), *itis* (inflammation), and thus, inflammation around the heart. Substitute the prefix *dys-* before menorrhea, *dys* (disordered), *meno* (menstrual), *rrhea* (discharge); hence, a painful or difficult menstruation. Gastroenterostomy: *gastro* (stomach), *enter* (intestine), *ostomy* (surgical opening), would mean a surgical opening from the stomach into the intestine. (L and G stand for Latin and Greek, respectively.)

A, AB- ABS- (L) From, away; departing from the normal.

AD- (L) Addition to, toward, nearness; adduct, to draw toward a center.

AMB- , AMBI- (L) Both; ambidextrous, having the ability to work effectively with either hand.

AMPHI- (G) On both sides; amphiarthrosis, form of articulation permitting little motion; amphibolic, uncertain.

AMPHO- (G) Both; amphodiplopia, double vision in both eyes.

AN- (G) Negative, without or not; anacid, lacking in acidity.

ANA- (G) Up, back again; anabiosis, a restoration after apparent death.

ANDRO- (G) Signifying man; androgen, a substance producing or stimulating male characteristics.

ANTE- (L) Front, before; antefebrile, before the onset of fever.

ANTERO- (L) Front, before; anterolateral, before and to one side.

ANTHROPO- (G) Denoting man; anthropology, the science that treats of man.

ANTI- , ANT- (G) Against; antibiotic, to destroy bacteria.

APO- (G) Away, separation; apocrine, cells which lose part of their cytoplasm while functioning.

ARCH- , ARCHE- , ARCHI- (G) Beginning; archetype, primitive type form from which other forms have developed by differentiation.

ARSENO- (G) Denoting the chemical group; arsenotherapy, the treatment of disease with arsenic preparations.

ARYL- Denoting a radical of the aromatic series; arylarsonate, salt of arylarsonic acid.

ATELO- (G) Imperfect development. Atelocheilia, imperfect development of the lip; harelip.

AZO- (G) Denoting a substance from a hydrocarbon being replaced by nitrogen of a portion of the hydrogen; azonic, that which contains no living organisms.

BARO- (G) Weight; baromachrometer, the instrument used for weighing and measuring infants at birth.

BARY- (G) Heavy, dull, hard; baryglossia, having a slow utterance of speech.

BILI- (L) Pertaining to bile; biliation, the secretion of bile.

BRADY- (G) Denoting slow; bradycardia, abnormally slow heart beat; bradycrotic, a slow pulse.

BROM- , BROMO- (L) A stench; Bromidrosis, offensive perspiration.

BRONCHO- (G) Relating to the bronchi; bronchoadenitis, inflammation of the bronchial glands.

CAC- (G) Bad; cachexia, a state of ill health, malnutrition and wasting.

CARDIO- (G) Relating to the heart; cardiocentesis, a surgical puncture of the heart.

CARPO- (G) Pertaining to the carpus; carpoptosis, a falling, wrist drop.

CATA- (G) Down or downward; against; catacleisis, closure of eyelids by spasm or adhesion.

CERVICO- (L) Relating to the neck; cervicobrachial, the neck and arm.

CARDI- , CARDIO- (G) Relating to the heart; cardiectasia, dilation of the heart.

CINESI- (G) Denoting motion; cinesia, seasickness; cinesthesia, the sensation of motion.

CIRCA- (L) About; circulation, movement in a circular course.

CIRCUM- (L) Around; circumarticular, surrounding a joint.

CON- (L) Together with; concavity, a hollow surface with curved sides.

CONTRA- (L) Opposite, against; contra-aperture, a second opening made in an abscess.

CUNEO- (L) A wedge; cuneocuboid, pertaining to cuboid and cuneiform bones, those of the tarsus, sole of foot and edge of eyelid.

CO- (L) Signifying with or together; coalescence, the fusion or blending of parts.

DECI- (L) Denoting tenth.

DEMI- (L) Meaning half; demilune, half-moon shaped cells.

DI- (G) Twice; diagnostic, said of symptoms.

DIALY- (G) To separate, dialysis, the passage of diffusible substances through a membrane.

DIA- (G) Meaning through; diadermic, through the skin.

DIAZO- (G) Possession of the group N^2; diazomethane, an extremely poisonous yellow gas, used in organic synthesis.

DIS- (G) Apart, duplication, separation; disacidify, the removal of an acid from a mixture.

DOLICHO- (G) Meaning long; dolichocolon, having an abnormally long colon.

ECTO- (G) On the outside, without; ectocondyle, an external condyle of a bone; ectopic, out of the normal place.

EN- (G) Meaning in; encysted, surrounded by membrane.

END- , ENDO- (G) Denoting inward, within; endoaortitis, inflammation of the inner coat of the aorta.

ENTO- (G) Within, inner; entotic, arising within the ear.

EPI- , EP- (G) On or upon, in addition to; epigastrium, region over the pit of the stomach.

EX- (L.) Out, away from; exanthematous, pertaining to an eruption or rash.

EXO- (L) Without, outside of; exophthalmos, pertaining to the protrusion of the eyeball.

EXTRA- (L) Outside of; in addition to; extradural, on outer side of the dura mater.

FIBRO- (L) Relating to fibers; fibroblastoma, a tumor of connective tissue.

FORE- (O.E.) Before or in front of; forearm,

the part of the arm between the elbow and the wrist.

FRONTO- (L) Pertaining to front; fronto-parietal, relating to the frontal and parietal bones.

FERRI- , FERRO- (L) Indicating the presence of iron; ferrihemoglobin, a reduced form of hemoglobin.

GASTER- , GASTR- , GASTRO- (G) Pertaining to the stomach; gastroenterostomy, a surgical opening between the stomach and intestines.

HEMI- (G) Meaning half; hemicrania, unilateral head pain, usually migraine.

HEMO- (G) Relating to the blood; hemoptysis, expectoration of blood arising from hemorrhage of the lung.

HEPAT-, HEPATICO-, HEPATO- (G) Pertaining to the liver; hepatitis, inflammation of the liver.

HEREDO- (L) Relating to heredity; heredoataxia, hereditary lack of order.

HEX-, HEXA- (G) Meaning six; hexa-vaccine, a vaccine made from six different microorganisms.

HETER-, HETERO- (G) Meaning other, relationship to another; heterochromia, a diversity of color.

HOMEO- (G) Denoting likeness or resemblance; homeostasis, the state of relative constancy of the body fluids.

HOMO- (G) Denoting sameness; homologous, similar in fundamental structure and in origin, but not necessarily in function.

HYAL-, HYALO- (G) Transparent; hyaloid, glassy.

HYPER- (G) Denoting above, excessive or beyond; hyperchylia, the abnormal secretion of gastric juice.

HYPO- (G) Below, less than; hypodermic, insertion under the skin, as a hypodermic injection.

IDEO- (G) Pertaining to mental images; ideophrenic, having abnormal ideas of a perverted nature.

IDIO- (G) Denoting relationships to one's self or to something separate and distinct; idiopathic, self originated.

IN- (L) Not, in, inside, within; also intensive action; inarticulate, without joints.

INFRA- (L) Below; infrascapular, beneath the shoulder blade.

INTER- (L) In the midst, between; inter-femoral, between the thighs.

INTRA- (L) Denoting within; intracutaneous, within the substance of the skin.

INTRO- (L) Denoting in or into; introvert, to dwell within one's self, thus withdrawing from reality, and external environment.

ISCHIO- (G) Pertaining to the ischium; ischioneuralgia, pain in the hip; synonymous with sciatica.

ISO- (G) Denoting equal, or alike; isochromatic, having the same color.

JUXTA- (L) Of close proximity; juxtaposition, adjacent, or side by side, continuity, in immediate succession.

KARYO- (G) Relating to a cell's nucleus; karyolymph, fluid in the meshes of the nucleus.

KAT-, KATA- (G) Down; katachromiasis, breaking down process of chromosomes.

KENO- (G) Meaning empty; kenophobia, having a morbid fear of wide open spaces.

KETO- (G) Relating to the carbonyl group; CO; ketogenesis, the production of acetone bodies.

KILO- (G) Denoting 1,000; kilocycle, the frequency of 1,000 cycles per second.

KYPHO- (G) Denoting humped; kyphosis, spinal curvature.

LARYNGO- (G) Pertaining to the larynx; laryngology, the practice of medicine dealing with the treatment of diseases of the larynx.

LONG- (L) Meaning long; longevity, length of life.

MEDI- (L) The middle; medial, pertaining to the middle.

MESO- (G) Denoting middle; mesoderm, the middle layer of the germ layers.

METOPO- (G) Denoting forehead; metopodynia, frontal headache.

MILLI- (L) Meaning 1000 of a part: milligram, the unit of weight in the metric system.

MYELO- (G) The spinal cord, or bone marrow; myelography, a roentgenographical study of the spinal cord.

OARI-, OARIC- (G) Pertaining to the ovary; oaritis, inflammation of an ovary.

OB- (L) Denoting towards, against, in the way of; obesity, having an abnormal amount of fat on the body.

OMNI- (L) Meaning all; omnipotent, almighty, infinite in power; as God is omnipresent, present everywhere at the same time.

PER- (L) Meaning through, by means of; peracidity, abnormal acidity.

PERI- (G) Around, about, periarterial, placed around an artery.

PHACO- (G) Pertaining to lens of the eye; phacocystectomy, surgical excision of part of the crystalline lens capsule for cataract.

POST- (L) Meaning behind or after; postclavicular, located behind the clavicle (collarbone).

POSTERO- (L) Relating to the posterior; posterolateral, that which is located behind and at the side of a part.

PRE- (L) Meaning before; precancerous, taking place before the development of a carcinoma.

PRO- (L & G) Before, in front of; prognosis, prediction of course and end of a disease.

PSEUDO- (G) Denoting false; pseudocrisis, a false crisis.

RE- (L) Back, again (contrary); reaction, response to a stimulus.

RETRO- (L) Meaning backward; retroflexion, bending backwards.

SEMI- (L) Meaning half; seminormal, one half the normal standard.

SESQUI- (L) Meaning one and a half.

SKELETO- (G) Denoting skeleton; skeletogenous, forming skeletal structures.

STEATO- (G) Meaning fatty; steatopathy, disease of the sebaceous glands of the skin.

SUB- (L) Under, near; subcutaneous, located beneath the skin.

SYN- (G) Meaning joined together; synchronism, events occurring simultaneously.

THIO- (L) Denoting presence of sulfur replacing oxygen; thiopexy, the fixation of sulfur.

TRANS- (L) Meaning across, over; transection, cutting across a section.

TRI- (G & L) Denoting three; triad, any trivalent element in chemistry; triangle, an area formed by 3 angles and 3 sides.

ULTRA- (L) Denoting beyond, excess; ultraligation, ligation of a blood vessel beyond the origin of a branch.

UN- (A.S.) Meaning not, reversal; unciform, hook-shaped; unconscious, state of being without consciousness.

SUFFIXES

-ABLE, -IBLE, -BLE (L) The power to be, as inevitable.

-AD (L) Meaning toward, in the direction of.

-AGE (L) Put in motion, to do; massage.

-AGRA (L) A seizure; a severe pain.

-ALGIA (G) Denoting pain. Cephalgia, pain in the head.

-AEMIA (G) Pertaining to blood.

-ASE (L) A suffix forming the name of an enzyme; lipase.

-BLAST (G) Designates a cell or a structure.

-CELE (G) Denoting a swelling. Enterocele, a hernia of the intestine.

-CENTESIS (G) Denoting puncture. Thoracentesis, a surgical puncture of the chest.

-ECTOMY (G) A cutting out. Pneumonectomy, a removal of a lung.

-EMIA (G) Denoting blood. Anemia, a deficiency of quantity and quality of blood.

-ESTHESIA (G) Denoting sensation. Anesthesia, the loss of feeling or sensation.

-FACIENT (L) Indicating that which makes or causes.

-GENE; -GENESIS; -GENETIC; -GENIC (G) Denoting production, origin. Bronchogenic, originating in the lung.

-GOG; -GOGUE (O.F.) To make flow.

-GRAM (G) A tracing; a mark. Electrocardiogram, a graphic tracing of the action of the heart (EKG, ECG).

-GRAPH (G) A writing; a record. Encephalography, a graphic examination of the brain.

-IASIS (G) Condition, pathological state. Lithiasis, an existing calculi.

-ID (G) Denoting shape, or resembling, resemblance.

-IDAE (L) Forms the scientific names of zoological families; canidoe (the Oog family).

-IDE (L) Indicating a binary compound; as sodium chloride.

-ITE (G) Denoting of the nature of.

-ITIS (G) The significance of inflammation. Enterocolitis, inflammation of the small intestine and colon.

-LOGIA (G) Denoting discourse, science or study of. Neurology, the study of the nervous system.

-OID (G) Denoting form of, resemblance. Carcinoid, a tumor in stomach.

-OMA (G) Denoting a tumor. Carcinoma, a malignant new growth.

-OSIS (G) Denoting any morbid process or increase, physiologic or pathologic osteomiosis, disintegration of bone.

-OSTOMOSIS, -OSTOMY (G) An outlet, to furnish with a mouth. Duodenostomy, a surgical opening into the duodenum.

-PLASTY (G) Indicates molding or shaping.

-RHAGIA (G) Denoting a discharge; usually a bleeding.

-RHAPHY (G) Meaning suturing or stitching.

-RHEA (G) Meaning to flow; indicates discharge.

-SCOPY (G) Generally indicating an instrument for viewing.

-STOMY (G) To furnish with an opening, mouth.

-TOMY (G) Denoting a cutting operation.

-TROPHY (G) Denoting a relationship to nourishment.

-YL (G) Denoting chemistry, a radical.

-YLENE (G) Denoting in chemistry a bivalent hydrocarbon radical.

COMBINING FORMS

AER-, AERO- (G) Denoting air or gas; aerated, containing air or gas.

ALGE-, ALGESI-, ALGO-, (G) Relating to pain; algogenic, that which causes neuralgic pain. Algesic, painful.

ALLO- (G) Other, differing from the normal; allochroism, to change in color.

ALLOTRIA- (G) Strange or foreign; allotriophagy, a craving for unusual foods.

AMYLO- (G) Relating to starch; amylogenic, the producing of starch.

ANOMALO- (G) Irregularity; anomaly, a marked deviation from the normal.

ANTHRACO- (G) Relating to coal, also carbon dioxide; anthracosis, a condition of the pulmonary organs caused by inhaling coal dust.

ANTRO- (L) Relating to the antrum or sinuses; antrocele, accumulated fluid in the maxillary antrum.

ARRHENO- (G) Denoting male; arrhenogenic, the production of male offspring only.

ARTHRO- (G) Relating to a joint or joints; arthrodesis, a surgical fixation of a joint by fusion of the joint surfaces.

ATMO- (G) Relating to vapor; atmograph, the recording of respiratory movements.

ATRETO- (G) Denoting closed; atretocystia, a closure of the bladder.

AUXO- (G) Growth, acceleration; auxocardia, an enlargement of the heart.

AXIO- (L & G) Relating to an axis; axion, the brain and spinal cord.

BREPHO- (G) Denoting embryo or fetus; brephotrophic, the nourishment of infants.

BREVI- (L) Short, brevicollis, having a short neck.

CELIO- (G) Denoting the abdomen; celiogastrotomy, an incision of the stomach through an abdominal section.

CENTRO- (G) Center; centrostaltic, relating to the center of motion.

CHEILO-, CHEIL- (G) Denoting lip; cheilocarcinoma, cancer of the lip.

CHEIRO-, CHEIR- (G) Relating to the hand; cheirospasm, writer's cramp.

CHEMO- (G) Relating to a chemical; chemomorphosis, a change of form due to chemical action.

CHIRO-, CHIR- (G) Denoting hand; chirognomy, the study of the hand as a guide to character; chiromegaly, enlargement of the hands.

CHLORO- (G) Denoting green; chloropane, green-yellow pigment in the retina.

CHOLE-, CHOL-, CHOLO- (G) Relating to the bile; cholecystitis, inflammation of the gallbladder.

CHONDR-, CHONDRI- (G) Relating to cartilage; chondrocostal, pertaining to the ribs and costal cartilages.

CHROM-, CHROMO- (G) Relating to color; chromocyte, any colored cell.

CIRSO- (G) Relating to a varix; cirsodesis, the ligation of varicose veins.

CLEIDO-, CLEID- (G) Denoting clavicle; cleidocostal, pertaining to the clavicle and ribs.

COLEO-, COLE- (G) Denoting a sheath; relating to the vagina; coleoptosis, prolapse of the vagina.

COLPO-, COLP- (G) Relating to the vagina; colpocystotomy, a surgical incision into the bladder through the vagina.

COPRO- (G) Denoting feces; coprostasis, constipation.

CRANIO- (L) Cranium of the skull; cranioclasis, an operation of crushing of the fetal head; craniopathy, any disease of the skull.

CRYMO- (G) Denoting cold; crymoanesthesia, refrigeration anesthesia.

CRYO- (G) Relating to cold; cryogenic, producing low temperatures. Cryosurgery, the cryosurgeons tool is a silver-tipped, hollow probe, chilled by liquid nitrogen, thus replacing the scalpel in some major surgery.

CYSTO- (G) Relating to a sac, or cyst; cystofibroma, fibroma containing cysts.

CRYPT- (G) To hide, a pit; cryptoglioma, a glioma that has not revealed itself.

CYTO- (G) Denoting the cell; cytohistogenesis, the structural development of the cell.

CYANO- (G) Denoting dark blue; cyanosis, bluish coloring of the skin.

CYCLO- (G) Pertaining to a cycle; cycloid, an extreme variation of moods, from elation to melancholia.

CYNO- (G) Denoting dog; cynophobia, having a morbid fear of dogs.

DACTYLO- (G) Relating to digits, fingers or toes; dactylography, a study of fingerprints.

DACRYO- (G) Pertaining to the lachrymal glands; dacryocystitis, inflammation of the tear sac (involving mucous membrane of the lacrimal sac.)

DEC-, DECA- (G) Ten; decagram, 10 grams in weight.

DENTO-, DENT- (L) Relating to teeth; dentoid, tooth shaped.

DERMA-, DERMAT- (G) Relating to the skin; dermatoconiosis, any skin irritation caused by dust, an occupational dermatitis.

DESMO- (G) Relating to a bond, or ligament; desmodynia, pain in a ligament.

DEUTERO-, DEUTO- (G) Meaning second. Deuteropathic, occurring secondarily to some other diseases.

DEXTRO- (L) Right; dextrocerebral, the right side of the brain being more active than the left.

DIPLO- (G) Double, twofold; diplopia, having double vision.

DORSI-, DORSO- (L) Referring to the back; dorsiflection, bending backward.

DROMO- (G) Denoting running; dromomania, having a mania for roaming.

DUODENO- (L) Relating to the duodenum; duodenojejunostomy, a surgical formation of a communication between the duodenum and the jejunum.

DYNAMO- (G) Denoting power or strength; dynamo genesis, the ability to put forth increased energy.

ECHINO- (G) Denoting relationship to spines; echinococcous, a type of tapeworm, small in size.

ELECTRO- (G) Relating to electricity; electrocautery, the cauterizing of tissue by means of an electric current.

ELEO- (G) Denoting relationship to oil; eleoma, a tumor caused by injection of oil into the tissues.

ENCEPHALO- (G) Denoting the brain; encephalography, a roentgenogram examination of the brain.

ENTERO- (G) Relating to the intestines; enteropexy, the union of divided parts of the intestines; enterorrhexis, rupture of the intestines.

EPISIO- (G) Relating to the vulva; episiorrhaphy, suturing of the labia majora.

ERGO- (G) Relating to work; ergodermatosis, an occupational dermatitis.

EROTO- (G) Relating to love, or sexual desire; erotology, the study of love; erotogenic, producing sexual excitement.

ESO- (G) Inward; esophagodynia, having pain in the esophagus.

ESTHESIO- (G) Relating to feeling or sensation; esthesioneurosis, having any disorder of the sensory nerves.

FACIO- (L) Relating to the face; facioplegia, having facial paralysis.

GAMETO- (G) Relating to a gamete; gametogenesis, development of the male and female sex cells.

GANGLIO-, GANGLI (G) Relating to a ganglion; gangliocytoma, a tumor which contains ganglion cells.

GENI- (G) Relating to the chin; geniohyoid, relating to the chin and hyoid bone.

GENO- (G) Relating to reproduction; genotype, hereditary constitution of an individual.

GENU- (L) Relating to the knee. Genupectoral, relating to the knee and chest.

GERO-, GERONTO- (G) Denoting old age; gerontology, the study of the aged.

GIGANTO- (G) Meaning huge; gigantocyte, a very large red blood corpuscle.

GINGIVO- (L) The gingiva, or gum; gingivoglossitis, inflammation of the gums and tongue.

GLIO- (G) Denoting a glue-like substance; glioma, a tumor composed of neuroglia cells.

GLOSSO-, GLOSS- (G) Relating to the tongue; glossitis, inflammation of the tongue.

GLUCO- (G) Denoting sweetness; glucogenic, producing glucose, a sweet substance.

GLYCO- (G) Relating to sugar; glycohemia, having sugar in the blood.

GNATHO-, GNATH- (G) Denoting the jaw; gnathodynia, pain in the jaw.

GON- (G) Denoting seed; gonad, an ovary or testis; (a gamete-producing gland).

GONIO- (G) Denoting an angle; gonion, the tip of the angle of the jaw.

GONY- (G) Relating to the knee; gonyectyposis, bowleg.

GRAPHO- (G) Denoting writing; graphology, an examination of handwriting, as a means of diagnosis in diseases of the nerves.

GYMO- (G) Denoting nakedness; gymnosophy, nudism.

GYRO- (G) Denoting gyrus; gyrose, marked by circles or curved lines.

HALO- (G) Denoting salt; haloid, saltlike.

HAMART-, HAMARTO- (G) Relating to a defect; hamartoma, a tumor-like nodule.

HAPLO- (G) Denoting single, or simple; haplopathy, an uncomplicated disease; haplont, a single individual.

HAPT-, HAPTE-, HAPTO- (G) Relating to touch or to seizure; haptometer; an instrument used to measure the sensitivity to touch.

HELICO- (G) Relating to a snail, or a coil; helicopodia, a snail like gait.

HELO- (G) Relating to a nail, or to a callus; heloma, a corn on a toe.

HIER-, HIERO- (G) Relating to the sacrum; hierolisthesis, displacement of the sacrum.

HISTIO-, HISTO-, HIST- (G) Relating to tissue; histoclastic, a breaking down of tissue.

HOLO- (G) Relating to the whole; holotonia, a muscular spasm enveloping the whole body.

HYDR-, HYDRO- (G) Denoting water; hydrocephalus, an abnormal accumulation of fluid on the cranial vault.

HYGRO- (G) Denoting moisture; hygroscopic, the absorption of moisture.

HYL-, HYLE-, HYLO- (G) Denoting matter, material, hylotropic, the change of form without change of composition, as from vapor to liquid.

HYPSO- (G) Relating to height; hypsophobia, a fear of great heights.

IATRO- (G) Relating to medicine; iatrology, the science of medicine.

ICHTHYO- (G) Relating to fish; ichthyosis, a scaliness of the skin (due to hypertrophy of the horny layer).

ILEO-, ILIO- (L) Relating to the ileum; ileocolitis, inflammation of the ileum and the cecum.

INO- (G) Relating to fibrous material; inochondritis, inflammation of a fibrocartilage.

IPSI- (L) (Meaning self); relating to same; ipsilateral, pertaining to the same side.

IRIDO- (G) Relating to a colored circle; iridodilator, dilatation of the pupils.

ISO- (G) Meaning equal; isocellular, composed of equal and similar cells.

JEJUNO- (L) Referring to the jejunum, jejunoileostomy, formation of a passage between the jejunum and the ileum.

KERATO- (G) Relating to cornea; keratocentesis, corneal puncture.

KINO- (G) Denoting movement; kinotome, an instrument for measuring the degree of motion.

KOILO- (G) Denoting concave, or hollow; koilorrhachic, curvature of the spine with a forward concavity.

LABIO- (L) Pertaining to the lips; labiogingival, relating to the lips and gums.

LACTO- (L) Relating to milk; lactogenic, stimulating milk production.

LALO- (G) Pertaining to speech; (laloneuroses, a nervous speech disorder); lalorrhea, an excessive flow of words.

LAPARO- (G) Pertaining to the loin or flank; laparotomy, surgical opening of the abdomen.

LATERO- (L) Pertaining to the side; lateroversion, turning to one side.

LEIDO-, LEIO- (G) Denoting smooth; leidermia, abnormally smooth skin.

LEPIDO- (G) Denoting flake, or scale; lepidosis, a scaly eruption.

LEUKO-, LEUK (G) Denoting deficiency of color; leukocyte, white blood corpuscle.

LIENO- (L) Denoting the spleen; lienopancreatic, pertaining to both the spleen and pancreas.

LIP-, LIPO- (G) Pertaining to fat; lipoblastoma, a tumor of fatty tissue.

LITHO- (G) Denoting a calculus; lithonephrotomy, the surgical removal of a renal calculus.

MACR-, MACRO- (G) Meaning large, long; macropodia, having large feet.

MALACO- (G) Denoting softness; malacoplakia, the formation of soft patches on the mucuous membrane of a hollow organ; malacosarcosis, softness of muscular tissue.

MASTRO-, MAST- (G) Relating to the breast; mastodynia, pain in the breast.

MEG-, MEGA- (G) Denoting great, large; megacephalic, having an abnormally large head.

MELI- (G) Meaning sweet; melicera, viscid or syrupy substance.

MENINGO- (G) Denoting membranes; covering the brain and spinal cord; meningomyelitis, inflammatory condition of the spinal cord.

MERO- (G) Combining form denoting part; merocoxalgia, painful condition of the thigh and hips.

METRA-, METRO- (G) Relating to the uterus; metroptosis, a prolapse of the uterus.

MICR-, MICRO- (G) Denoting small size, extent; microsthenic, having weak muscular power.

MITO- (G) Relating to thread, threadlike; mitosis, the indirect division of cells.

MOGI- (G) Denoting difficulty; mogilalia, stuttering.

MONO- (G) Denoting one; monochroic, of one color.

MORPHO- (G) Relating to form; morphology, that part of biology which deals with structure and form.

MULTI- (L) Denoting many; multigravida, having three or more pregnancies.

MYC-, MYCET- (G) Denoting fungus; mycosis, a fungus disease.

MY-, MYO- (G) Relating to muscle; myocardial, pertaining to the muscular tissue of the heart.

MYRINGO- (L) Denoting tympani, or eardrum; myringotomy, a surgical incision of the membrana tympani.

MYX-, MYXO- (G) Pertaining to mucus; myxofibroma, a tumor consisting of mucous and fibrous elements.

NANO- (L) Denoting smallness; nanomelia, having abnormally small limbs.

NARCO- (G) Denoting stupor; narcolepsy, an uncontrollable desire for sleep.

NASO- (L) Relating to the nose; naso-oral; pertaining to both the nose and the mouth.

NECRO- (G) Denoting death; necrology, the recording of deaths.

NEMATO- (G) Denoting a threadlike structure; nematoda, meaning worms.

NEO- (G) Denoting new; neonatal, a newly born infant.

NEPHELO- (G) Denoting cloudiness; nephelopia, cloudiness of the cornea.

NEPHRO-, NEPHR- (G) Denoting kidney; nephrosclerosis, a hardening of the kidney.

NITRO- (G) Denoting presence of nitrogen; nitrofurazone, a synthetic antibiotic for topical application (in some skin diseases).

NOMO- (G) Denoting usage, or law; nomogenesis, the theory of evolution fixed or predetermined by law.

NORMO- (L) Denoting normal or usual; normoglycemia, having a normal amount of sugar in the blood.

NOSO- (G) Denoting disease; nosology, the classification of diseases.

NOTO- (G) Relating to the back; notomyelitis, an inflammation of the spinal cord.

NUDI- (L) Denoting uncovered, naked; nudomania, abnormal desire to be nude.

NYCTO- (G) Denoting night or darkness; nyctohemeral, both day and night.

NYMPHO- (G) Relating to the nymphae;

nymphotomy, a surgical incision of the nymphae or clitoris.

OCULO- (L) Denoting the eye; oculomotor, relating to the movements of the eye.

ODYNO- (G) Denoting pain; odynophagia, painful swallowing of food.

OLEO- (L) Denoting oil; oleovitamin, solution of vitamin and oil combination.

OMO- (G) Relating to the shoulder; omodynia, pain of the shoulder.

OMPHAL-, OMPHALO- (G) Relating to the naval; omphalitis, inflammation of the umbilicus.

ONCO- (G) Denoting swelling or mass; oncolysis, destruction of tumor cells.

ONEIRO- (G) Relating to a dream; oneirodynia, a nightmare.

ONYCO- (G) Relating to the nails; onychocryptosis, ingrown toenail.

OO- (G) Denoting an egg; oocyte, the early or primitive ovum before it has developed completely.

OPISTH-, OPISTHO- (G) Denoting backward; opisthotonos, denoting tetanic spasm in which the head and heels are bent backward and the body bowed forward.

OPHTHAL-, OPHTHALMO- (G) Pertaining to the eye; ophthalmomyositis, inflamed condition of the eye muscles.

OPTICO- (G) Relating to the eye or vision; opticopupillary, concerning the optic nerve and the pupil.

OPTO- (G) Denoting vision or sight; (optostriate, concerning the optic thalamus and the corpus striatum); optometrist, one who fits glasses to correct ocular defects (measures the refractive powers, the degree of visual acuity).

ORO- (L) Relating to the mouth; orolingual, relating to the mouth and the tongue.

ORCHI-, ORCHO- (G) Relating to the testes; orchidectomy, removal of a testicle.

ORTHO- (G) Meaning straight, or right; orthopedics, the correction of deformities.

OSCHEO- (G) Denoting the scrotum; oscheoma, a tumor of the scrotum.

OSCILLO- (L) Denoting oscillation; oscillopsia, having oscillating vision, objects moving back and forth.

OSMO- (G) Denoting odor; osmodysphoria, abnormal dislike of certain odors. Denoting relationship to osmosis, passage of a solution through a membrane.

OSTEO- (G) Relating to the bones; osteoarthritis, a disease of the bones with joint involvement.

OTO-, OT- (G) Denoting the ear; otocleisis, a closure of the auditory passages.

OVARIO- (G) Denoting the ovary; ovarioectomy, removal of an ovary.

OVI-, OVO- (L) Denoting an egg; ovogenesis, the production of ova.

OXY- (G) Denoting sharp, keen; oxycephalia, having a high and pointed skull.

PACHY-, PACH- (G) Meaning thick, large, heavy; pachycephalic, possessing a thick skull.

PALATO- (L) Denoting the palate; palotoplasty, repair of a cleft palate.

PALI-, PALIN- (G) Denoting again, or a pathologic repetition; palindromia, a recurrence of a disease.

PATHO- (G) Denoting disease; pathological, relating to the onset of a disease.

PEDIA-, PEDO- (G) Denoting child; pediatrics, the branch of medicine which treats the child and its development.

PENTA-, PENT- (G) Meaning five. Pentachromic, capable of distinguishing only five colors.

PERINEO- (G) A combining form for region between anus and the scrotum or the vulva; perineorrhaphy, suturing of the perineum, performed for the repair of a laceration.

PERO- (G) Denoting deformed, or maimed; perobrachius, a fetus with deformed arms.

PERONEO- (G) Pertaining to the fibula; peroneus, one of three muscles of the leg causing motion in the foot.

PHAGO- (G) Denoting relationship to eating; phagomania, an insatiable craving for food.

PHANER-, PHANERO- (G) Meaning evident, visible; phanerosis, the process of becoming visible.

PHARYNGO- (G) Pertaining to the pharynx; pharyngoparalysis, paralysis of the muscles of the pharynx.

PHLEB-, PHLEBO- (G) Denoting the veins; phlebogenous, formation in the veins.

PHLOGO- (G) Denoting inflammation; phlogotic, inflammatory.

PHON-, PHONO- (G) Denoting sound; phonocardiograph, recording the sounds of the heart.

PHOT-, PHOTO- (G) Relating to light; photodysphoria, intolerance to light.

PHREN- (G) Relating to the mind; phrenesthesia, feeble mindedness.

PHYSIO- (G) Denoting nature; physiognosis, diagnosis determined from one's facial expression and appearance of the eyes.

PHYSO- (G) Relating to air or gas; physometra, air or gas in the uterine cavity.

PHYT-, PHYTO- (G) Meaning a plant, or that which grows; phytosis, any disease of vegetable parasitic origin.

PICR-, PICRO- (G) Meaning bitter; picroglossia, having a bitter taste.

PILO- (L) Denoting hair; pilosebaceous, relating to hair glands and sebaceous glands.

PIMELO- (G) Denoting fat; pimelosis, obesity.

PIO- (G) Denoting fat; pionemia, blood which contains oil or fat.

PLASMO- (G) Relating to plasma, or substance of a cell; plasmosome, a cell having a true nucleus.

PLATY- (G) Meaning broad or flat; platycnemia, platycnemism; having an unusually broad tibia; broadlegged.

PNEUMA-, PNEUMONO-, PHEUMOTO- (G) Denoting air or gas; pneumocentesis, paracentesis or surgical puncture of a lung.

POD-, PODO- (G) Meaning foot. Pododynia, pain in the feet.

POLIO- (G) Relating to the gray matter of the nervous system; polioencephalitis, a disease of the gray substance of the brain.

POLY- (G) Denoting many; polyarthritis, inflammation of a number of joints.

PROCT-, PROCTO- (G) Denoting the anus and rectum; proctologist, a specialist in diseases of the anus and rectum.

PROSO- (G) Denoting forward or anterior; prosopantritis, inflamed frontal sinuses.

PROSOPO- (G) Denoting the face; prosopoanochisis, an oblique facial cleft.

PROT-, PROTO- (G) Denoting first; protobrochal, the first stage of development of an ovary.

PSYCHO-, PSYCH- (G) Relating to the mind; psychosis, any mental disorder.

PTYALO- (G) Denoting the saliva; ptyalorrhea, an abnormal flow of saliva.

PUBIO-, PUBO- (L) Denoting the pubic hair, pubic bone or region; pubiotomy, incision between the pubic bones in order to enlarge the pelvic passage, (facilitating the delivery of the fetus when pelvis is malformed.)

PULMO- (L) Denoting lung; pulmonectomy, the removal of part or all of a lung.

PUPILLO- (L) Denoting the pupil; pupillotonia, a tonic reaction of the pupil, a failure to react to light.

PYCNO- (G) Denoting dense, thick; pycnosis, a thickening.

PYEL-, PYELO- (G) Denoting the pelvis; pyelocystitis, inflammation of the renal pelvis and the bladder.

PYLE- (G) Denoting orifice, especially that of the portal vein; pylemphraxis, occlusion of the portal vein.

PYLORO- (G) Relating to the pylorus (gatekeeper); pyloroduodenitis, inflammation of the mucosa of the pylorus and duodenum.

PY-, PYO- (G) Denoting pus; pyocelia, pus formation in the abdominal cavity.

PYRETO- (G) Denoting fever; pyretotyphosis, a delirious fever.

PYRO- (G) Denoting heat or fire; pyrosis, a burning sensation.

QUINTI- (L) Denoting five; quintisternal, the 5th bony portion of the sternum.

RACHI-, RACHIO- (G) Relating to the spine; rachianalgesia, spinal anesthesia.

RADIO- (L) Relating to radiation; radiodermatitis. Overexposure to roentgen rays causes inflammation of skin.

RECTO- (L) Denoting the rectum; rectoclysis, the slow introduction of fluid into the rectum.

RHABDO- (G) Denoting rod; rhabdomyoma, a striated muscular tissue tumor.

RHEO- (G) Denoting current, stream; rheostosis, a condition of hyperostosis marked by the presence of streaks in bones.

RHIN-, RHINO- (G) Denoting the nose; rhinocleisis, a nasal obstruction.

RHIZO- (G) Denoting root; rhizomelic, involving the hips and shoulders.

RRHAGIA- (G) Denoting abnormal discharge; hemorrhage.

SACCHARO- (G) Denoting sugar; saccharorrhea, the secretion of sugar in the body fluids, as in urine or perspiration.

SACRO- (L) Relating to the sacrum; sacrolumbar, pertaining to the sacrum and the loin.

SACTO- (G) Denoting stuffed; sactosalpinx,

dilated fallopian tube due to retention of secretions, as in pyosalpinx or hydrosalpinx.

SALPINGO- (G) Denoting a tube, specifically the fallopian tube; salpingo-oophorectomy, surgical excision of an oviduct and an ovary.

SAPRO- (G) Relating to decay; saprophyte, an organism living on decaying or dead organic matter.

SARCO.- (G) Denoting flesh; sarcoadenoma, a fleshy tumor of a gland.

SCAPHO- (G) Denoting boatlike; scaphocephalism, the condition of having a deformed head, projecting like the keel of a boat.

SCHISTO- (G) Denoting a split, or cleft; schistomelia, a cleft condition of a limb.

SCHIZO- (G) Denoting split; schizophrenia, a split personality.

SCIRRHO- (G) Denoting hard; scirrhosarca, hardening of the flesh, particularly of the new born.

SCHERO- (G) Denoting hardness; scleroderma, a thickening and hardening of the skin.

SCOLECO- (G) Denoting a worm; scolecoid, that which resembles a worm; a hydatid.

SCOLIO- (G) Denoting crooked, or twisting; scoliokyphosis, curvature of the spine.

SCOTO- (G) Relating to darkness; scotoma, a blind area in the visual field.

SERO- (L) Pertaining to serum; serocolitis, inflammation of the serous coat of the colon.

SIALO- (G) Relating to saliva or the salivary glands; sialoangitis, inflamed salivary ducts.

SIDERO- (G) Denoting iron; sideroderma, a bronzed coloration of the skin from disordered hemoglobin disintegration.

SINISTRO- (G) Denoting left; sinistrocerebral, located in the left cerebral hemisphere.

SITIO-, SITO- (G) Denoting bread, or made from grain; sitiology, the science of nutrition.

SOMATO- (G) Denoting the body; somatopsychic, both the body and the mind.

SOMNI- (L) Denoting sleep; somnipathis, one who is subject to hypnotic trance.

SPANO- (G) Denoting scarce or scanty; spanomenorrhea, scanty menstruation.

SPASMO- (L) Denoting a spasm; spasmolygmus, having spasmodic hiccups.

SPECTRO- (L) Denoting appearance, image; spectrocolorimeter, a device for detecting color blindness by isolating a single spectral color.

SPERMO-, SPERMATO- (G) Denoting sperm; spermatocele, a cystic tumor of the epididymis containing spermatozoa.

SPHENO- (G) Denoting wedge, the sphenoid bone (large bone at base of skull); sphenotresia, perforation of the skull in craniotomy.

SPHERO- (G) Denoting sphere, round; spherospermia, round spermatozoon, the mature male germ cell.

SPHYGMO- (G) Denoting pulse; sphygmopalpation, feeling of the pulse.

SPLEN-, SPLENO- (G) Denoting the spleen; splenocele, a hernia of the spleen.

SPODO- (G) Denoting waste materials; spodophorous, the removal of waste materials.

SPONDIO- (L) Spongelike; spongiosis, edema of the Malpighian (spongy layer) of the skin.

SPONDYLO- (G) Relating to the vertebrae or spinal column; spondylolisthesis, a forward partial dislocation of the lower lumbar vertebrae, usually on the sacrum resulting in pelvic deformity.

SPORO- (G) Denoting a spore; any germ; sporocyst, any cyst containing spores; sporogenesis, reproduction by spores.

STAPHYL-, STAPHYLO- (G) Resembling a bunch of grapes; staphylococcus, spherical, gram-positive bacteria.

STENO- (G) Denoting narrow, short, stenocoriasis, narrowing of the pupil of the eye.

STERCO- (L) Denoting feces; stercobilin, a brown pigment derived from the bile giving the characteristic color to feces.

STEREO- (G) Denoting solid; with three dimensions; stereo-cinefluorography, a photographic recording by motion picture camera of X-ray images produced by stereofluoroscopy, in three dimensional visualization.

STERNO- (G) Denoting sternum; sternocleidomastoid, one of two muscles arising from the sternum and inner part of the clavicle.

STETHO-, STETH- (G) Relating to the chest; stethoscope, an instrument used in auscultation or listening to the sounds produced in the body.

STHENO- (G) Denoting strength; sthenophotic, having the ability to see in a strong light.

STOMATO- (G) Denoting mouth; stomatorrhagia, hemorrhage from the mouth or gums.

STREPH-, STREPHO- (G) Denoting twisted; strephosymbolia, a disorder of perception.

STREPTO- (G) Denoting twisted; streptococcemia, presence of streptococci in the blood, causing infection.

STYLO- (L) Relating to a stylus or pointed instrument, stake-like; especially the styloid process; styloiditis, inflammation of the styloid process of the temporal bone.

SYM-, SYN- (G) Denoting with, along; synchronous, occurring at the same time; syndrome, a complex symptom.

TACHO-, TACHY- (G) Denoting swift; tachycardia, abnormal rapidity of heart action.

TARSO- (G) Relating to the flat of the foot; tarsoclasia, surgical fracture of the tarsus for correction of clubfoot.

TELO- (G) Denoting to an end; telotism, complete performance of a function; teleneuron, a nerve ending at which an impulse terminates.

TENO-, TENONTO- (G) Relating to a tendon; tenodesis, the suturing of the end of a tendon to a bone; tenontagra, a gouty infection of the tendons.

TERATO- (G) Denoting a marvel, prodigy, monster; teratoid, resembling a monster.

TERGO- (L) Denoting the back; tergolateral, pertaining to the back and side; also, dorsolateral.

TETRA-, TETR- (G) Denoting four; tetradactylous, having four fingers.

THALAMO- (G) Denoting chamber, that part of brain at which a nerve originates; thalamocortical, pertaining to the thalamus and the cerebral cortex.

THANATO- (G) Denoting death; thanatognomonic, indicative of the approach of death.

THERM-, THERMO- (G) Relating to heat; thermobiosis, the ability to withstand high temperature.

THORACO- (G) Relating to the chest, chest wall; thoracobronchotomy, a surgical incision through the thoracic wall into the bronchus.

THROMBO- (G) Denoting clot of blood; thromboangiitis, inflammation of the inner coat of blood vessel with clot formation.

THYMO- (G) Denoting the thymus gland; thymocyte, a lymphocyte-like cell having origin in the thymus gland.

THYREO-, THYRO- (G) Denoting oblong, shield, thyroid; thyreogenic, due to an excess or deficiency of the thyroid secretion.

TOCO- (G) Relating to childbirth; tocometer, an instrument for measuring the force of the uterine contractions in labor.

TOPO- (G) Denoting place; topography, a description of an anatomical region.

TOXICO-, TOXO- (G) Denoting poison; toxicohemia, blood poisoning. Toxicide, an agent which destroys a poison.

TRACHEO- (G) Denoting trachea, windpipe; tracheoesophageal, pertaining to the trachea and esophagus.

TRACHELO- (G) Denoting neck; trachelodynia, pain in the neck.

TRAUMATO- (G) Denoting trauma, an injury; traumatology, the study of wounds and their care.

TRICHI-, TRICHO- (G) Denoting hair; trichoclasis, brittle hair.

TYPHLO- (G) Denoting cecum; typhlomegaly, abnormal enlargement of the cecum.

TYRO- (G) Denoting cheese; tyroma, a caseous tumor, of a cheesy nature, or of cheesy matter.

UR-, URO-, URONO- (G) Relating to urine; urinary tract; uroclepsia, involuntary and unconscious discharge of urine.

VARICO- (L) Denoting twisting or swelling; varicosity, a swollen twisted vein.

VASO- (L) Denoting a vessel; vasoconstrictive, constriction of a blood vessel.

VENO- (L) Denoting a vein; venoperitoneostomy, the anastomosis of the saphenous vein with the peritoneum, permitting permanent drainage of the abdomen in ascites.

VENTRI-, VENTRO- (L) Denoting abdomen; front (anterior) aspect of the body; ventrovesicoflexion, a surgical operation in which the uterus is sutured to the bladder and abdominal wall.

VERTEBRO- (L) Relating to the vertebra; vertebronchondral, the vertebra and a costal cartilage.

VESICO- (L) Denoting bladder; vesicofixation, attachment of the uterus to the bladder, or the bladder to the abdominal wall.

VISCERO- (L) Denoting the organs of the body; viscerotomy, postmortem excision of a portion of the liver.

VIVI- (L) Denoting alive; vivisection, the cutting of or operation upon a living animal for physiological investigation and the study of disease.

XANTHO- (G) Denoting yellow; xanthochromia, a yellowish discoloration.

XERO- (G) Denoting dryness; xerocheilia, dry lips; exeroderma, roughness and dryness of the skin.

XIPHI-, XIPHO- (L) Denoting sword like in appearance; xiphocostal, xiphoid cartilage, cartilage shaped like a sword tip forming the lower extremity of the sternum and the ribs.

XYLO- (G) Denoting wood; xylosuria, the presence of xylose (wood sugar, a pentose) in the urine.

ZOO-, ZO- (G) Denoting animal; zoogenous, acquired from animals.

ZYGO- (G) Denoting yoke or joined; zygodactyly, the fusion of two or more fingers or toes.

ZYMO- (G) Denoting an enzyme, or to fermentation; zymolysis, digestion by means of an enzyme.

ABBREVIATIONS FREQUENTLY USED WITH SOME DERIVATIONS

Abbreviation	Definition with Derivation	Abbreviation	Definition with Derivation
A.A.L.	anterior axillary line	A.P.C.	auricular premature contraction
ab., ab	abortion; antibody	A.P. diameter	anteroposterior diameter
abd.; abd.	abdomen; abdominal	Aq.	water (*Aqua*, L)
Ab initio	from the beginning	Aq. com.	common water (*Aqua communis*, L)
a.c.	before meals (*ante cibos*, L)		
A.C., a.c.	air conduction (ear examination)	Aq. dest.	distilled water (*Aqua destillata*, L)
A.C.T.H.	adrenocorticotrophic hormone	Arg.	silver (*Argentum*, L)
ad	to; up to (*ad*, L)	A.S.	left ear; aortic stenosis
ad lib.	as desired (*ad libitum*, L)	A.S.D.	atrial or auricular septal defect
Adm.	admission	A.S.H.D.	arteriosclerotic heart disease
A.F.B.	Acid-fast bacilli	ASO	anti-streptolysin-O
A/G; A.G.	Albumin-globulin ratio (blood)	A-V	auriculoventricular or atrioventricular
A/J; A.J.	ankle jerk		
alb.	albumin, white	Av.	Avoirdupois (French)
Alt. die.	Alternate days (*Alternio die*, L)		
Alt. dieb.	Every other day (*Alternio diebus*, L)	BaEn.; BE	Barium enema
		BC.	bone conduction
Alt. hor.	Every other hour (*Alternis horis*, L)	Bib.	drink (*Bibe*, L)
		B.I.D.	twice a day (*Bis in die*, L)
Alt. noc.	Every other night (*Alternis noctus*, L)	B.I.N.	twice a night (*bis in noctus*, L)
		B.M.	bowel movement
amp.	ampule	B.M.R.; BMR	Basal metabolism rate
A₂	aortic second sound	BPH	benign prostatic hypertrophy
A₂, P₂	aortic second sound greater than pulmonic second	BRP	bathroom privileges
		BSP	bromsulphalein test
A/P, A.P.	anterior-posterior; anteroposterior; anteropituitary	B.U.N.	blood urea nitrogen

Abbreviation	Definition with Derivation	Abbreviation	Definition with Derivation
c̄	with (*cum*, *L*)	FBS	fasting blood sugar
C.	Centrigade (*Centrigadus*, *L*)	F.H.	Family History
C.	gallon (*Congius*, *L*)	Fld.	fluid (*fluidus*, *L*)
Cal.	calorie	fl. dr.	fluid dram (*fluidrachma*, *L*)
Cap.	capsule (*capsula*, *L*)	fl. oz.	fluid ounce (*fluidus uncia*, *L*)
C.B.C.	complete blood count	F.S.H.	follicle stimulating hormone
cc., c.c.	cubic centimeters	Ft., ft.	let there be made (*fiat*, *L*)
C.C.	chief complaint	FTLB	full-term living birth
C.F.T.	complement fixation test	FTND	full-term normal delivery
Cg.	Centrigram (French)	FUO	fever of undetermined origin
CHF	congestive heart failure		
cm	Centimeter (French)	GC	gonococcus, or gonococcal
CNS	central nervous system	G.I.	gastrointestinal
CO₂	carbon dioxide	gm.	gram (*gramme*, *French*)
Comp.	Compound (*Compositus*, *L*)	G.O.T.	glutemic oxyacetic trans-
Cong.	gallon, congenital (*Congitus*, *L*)		aminase
CR	cardiorespiratory	gr.	grain (*granum*, *L*)
CSF	cerebrospinal fluid	G.P.	General Practitioner
c.v.a.	costovertebral angle	G.P.I.	General paresis, or general
cysto.	cystoscopy		paresis of the insane.
		Gtt., gtt.	drops (*guttae*, *L*)
def.	defecation (*defaecatio*, *L*)	GTT	glucose tolerance test
diff.	differential (blood count)	GU	genitourinary
Dil., dil.	dilute, dilatation (OB) (*dilue*,	GYN	gynecology, -ical, -ist
	L)		
D.O.	Doctor of Osteopathy	H.	hour (*hora*, *L*)
DOA	dead on arrival	H.A.S.	hypertensive arterioscler -
DOE	dyspnea on exertion		otic
dr.	dram or drams (*drachma*, *L*)	Hb. or Hgb.	hemoglobin
DTR's	deep tendon reflexes	Hct.	hematocrit
DX	diagnosis	H.C.V.D.	Hypertensive cardiovascular
			disease
ECG, EKG	electrocardiogram	H. & E.	hemorrhage and exudate (eye)
EDC	expected date of confinement;	HEENT	head, ears, eyes, nose and
	estimated date of confine-		throat
	ment.	h.n.	tonight (*hac nocte*, *L*)
E.E.N.T.	eye, ear, nose and throat	hor. interm.	at intermediate hours (*horis*
elix.	elixir (Arabic)		*intermediis*, *L*)
emp.	emplastrum , a plaster	H.P.F., h.p.f.	high power field
E.N.T.	ear, nose and throat	h.s., H.S.	at bedtime or hour of sleep
ER.	epigastric region; Emergency		(*hora somni*, *L*)
	Room.	H.V.D.	hypertensive vascular disease
ESR	erythrocyte sedimentation rate	hypo	hypodermically (*hypo*, *Greek*:
EST	electroshock therapy		*under*)
ET	and (*et*, *L*)		
ext.	extract (extractum, *L*)	inf.	infusion (*infusum*, *L*) inferior
F.	Fahrenheit (*Proper name*, *L*)		
F.A.C.P.	Fellow, American College of	KC1	potassium chloride
	Physicians	KJ	knee jerk
F.A.C.S.	Fellow, American College of		
	Surgeons	l.	liter

Abbreviation	Definition with Derivation	Abbreviation	Definition with Derivation
L-1, L-2, etc.	First lumbar, second lumbar, etc.	N.P.	neuropsychiatry
		NPN	nonprotein nitrogen
lap.	laparotomy	N.R.	do not repeat
lat.	lateral	N.S.R.	normal sinus rhythm
Lb.	pound (*libra, L*)		
LBCD	left border of cardiac dullness	O.	pint (*Octavius, L*)
LCM	left costal margin	OB	Obstetrician, obstetrics
LE (prep.)	Lupus erythematous cell pre-paration	O.D., o.d.	right eye (oculus dexter)
		OH	occupational history
LH	lutenizing hormone	o.j.	orange juice
liq.	liquid; fluid (*liquor, L*)	ol.	oil (*Oleum, L*)
L.L.Q.	left lower quadrant	OLA	occiput left anterior
L.O.A.	left occipital anterior (occiput left anterior)	OLP	occiput left posterior
		omn. hor.	every hour (*omni hora, L*)
L.P.	lumbar puncture	omn. noct.	every night (*omni nocte, L*)
l/p.f.	lower power field	OPD	Outpatient department, clinic
L.P.V.	lymphopathia verereum	O.R.	Operating Room
LSK	liver, spleen and kidneys	os.	mouth, opening of cervix, *i.e.*, oscalis bone (*os; ora, L*)
L.U.L.	left upper lobe		
L.U.Q.	left upper quadrant	O.S., o.s.	left eye (oculus sinister)
LVE	left ventricular enlargement	O.U., o.u.	both eyes together, each eye
LVS	left ventricular strain	oz.	ounce (*uncia, L*)
LVH	left ventricular hypertrophy		
		P-231	radioactive phosphorus
M.	meter (French)	P-2	pulmonic second sound
m.	minimum (*minimum, L*)	PA	postero-anterior; pernicious anemia
M-1	mitral 1st sound		
MBC	maximum breathing capacity	P. & A.	percussion and auscultation
MCH	mean corpuscular hemoglobin	PAT	paroxysmal auricular tachy-cardia
MCHC	mean corpuscular hemoglobin concentration		
		PBI	protein bound iodine
M.C.L.	midclavicular line	p.c.	after food; after meals (*post cibum, L*)
MCV	mean corpuscular volume		
mEq/l	milliequivalents per liter	PCV	packed cell volume (blood) Hct.
MH	marital history		
mg. or mgm.	milligram	PDR	Physician's Desk Reference
MI	myocardial infarction; mitral insufficiency	P.E.	Physical examination
		PEG	pneumoencephalogram
mist.	mixture (*mistura, L*)	per	through or by
ml.	milliliter	PERRLA	pupils, equal, round, reactive to light and accommodation
mm.	millimeter (French)		
M.S.	multiple sclerosis; mitral steno-sis; morphine sulphate	P.H.	past history or personal history
		P.I.	present illness
MSL	midsternal line	P.I.D.	pelvic inflammatory disease
		pil.	pill (*pilula, L*)
n. b.	note well (*nota bene, L*)	P.I.P.	proximal interphalangeal joint
NBM, NPO		PMD	private medical doctor
(more common)	nothing by mouth	PMH	past medical history
no.	number (*numero, L*)	P.M.I.	point of maximum impulse
non rep.	don't repeat (*non repetatur, L*)	PND	paroxysmal night dyspnea
noxt.	at night (*nocte; noxte, L*)	P.o.	by mouth (*per os, L*)

Abbreviation	Definition with Derivation	Abbreviation	Definition with Derivation
P.P.D.	purified protein derivative, tuberculin test	R.O.T.	occiput right transverse
		R.Q.	respiratory quotient
P. physio.	physiotherapy; physical therapy	R.R.E.	round, regular and equal
		R.U.Q.	right upper quadrant
P.P.L.	Pleuropneumonia-like	R.U.L.	right upper lobe
pre-op	preoperative	R./x	take, prescription (*recipe, L*)
p.r.n.	as needed; as desired (*pro re nata, L*)		
P.S.P., PSP	phenosulfonphthalein tests	s̄	without (*sans, French*)
pt.	pint (*pinte, French*)	S.	mark (*signa, L*)
P.T.	physical therapy	SBE	shortness of breath on exertion
PTA	prior to admission	SBE	subacute bacterial endocarditis
puev.	powder (*pulvis, L*)		
P.U.R.	pyrexia of undetermined origin	S.c., Subq.	subcutaneously (*subcutis, L*)
P.V.C.	premature ventricular contraction	S.D.	septal defect
		SGO-T	serum glutamic oxalacetic transaminase
PZI	protamine zinc insulinate		
		SGP-T	serum glutamic pyruvic transaminase
q.d.	every day		
Q.h.	every hour (*quaque hora, L*)	SH	social history, serum hepatitis
Q₂h.	every two hours (*quaque hora, L*)		
		Sig.	let it be marked (*signetur, L*)
Q₃h.	every three hours (*quaque hora, L*))	S.O.B.	shortness of breath
		Sol.	solution (*solutio, L*)
q.i.d.	four times a day (*quater in die, L*)	s.o.s.	if occasion require, if necessary (*si opus sit, L*)
q.n.	every night	sp. gv.	specific gravity (*gravitus-heavy, L*)
qns	insufficient quantity		
q.o.d.	every other day	spt.	spirit (*spiritus, L*)
q.q.h.	every four hours	ss.	half (*semis, L*)
QRS	Ventricular wave on EKG	S.T.S.	serological test for syphillis
Q.s.	A sufficient quantity (*quantum sufficiat, L*)	stat.	immediately (*statim, L*)
		S.V.C.	superior vena cava
Qt.	quart (*quartina, L*)	syr.	syrup (*syrupus, L*)
quotid	daily (*quotidie, L*)		
Q.v.	as much as you will (*quantum vis, L*)	T.	temperature (*temperatura, L*)
		T. & A.	tonsillectomy and adenoidectomy
RAI	radioactive iodine		
RBBB	right bundle branch block	tab.	tablet (*tabella, L*)
RBC	red blood cells	t.i.d.	three times a day (*ter in die, L*)
RCM	right costal margin	t.i.n.	three times a night (*ter in nocte, L*)
Rh	Rhesus (monkey) factor in blood		
		TPR	temperature, pulse and respiration
rep.	let it be repeated (*repetatur, L*)		
R.L.L.	right lower lobe	T.U.R.	transurethral resection
R.L.Q.	right lower quadrant	tr., tinct.	tincture (*tinctura, L*)
R.M.L.	right middle lobe		
R.O.A.	occiput right anterior	Ua.	urinalysis
R.O.P.	occiput right posterior	ung.	ointment (*unguentum, L*)
R.O.S.	review of systems	Upper GI	upper gastrointestinal

Abbreviation	Definition with Derivation	Abbreviation	Definition with Derivation
Ur.	urine (*urina*, L)	VSD	ventricular septal defect
U.R.I.	upper respiratory infection		
U.S.P.H.S.	United States Public Health Service	WBC or wbc	white blood count
		w.d., or WD	well developed
		WF, WM	white female, white male
V.D.	venereal disease	w.n., or WN	well nourished
vin	wine (*vinum*, L)	Wt.	weight
Vol.%	volume per cent	WV	weight by volume

FREQUENTLY USED SYMBOLS

*	Birth	□, ♂	male
+	death	O, ♀	female
°	degree	#	number

TERMINOLOGY FREQUENTLY USED TO DESIGNATE BODY PARTS OR ORGANS

ANUS	Anal, ano	LIVER	Hepatic, hepato-
ARM	Brachial, brachio-	LUNGS	Pulmonary, pulmonic, pneumo
BLOOD	Hem, hemat-		
CHEST	Thoracic, thorax	MOUTH	Oral, os, stoma, stomat-
EAR	Auricle, oto-	MUSCLE	Myo-
EYE	Ocular, oculo-, Ophthalmo-	NECK	Cervix, cervical, cervico-
FOOT	Pedal, ped-, -pod	PENIS	Penile
GALLBLADDER	Chole, Chol-	RECTUM	Rectal
HEAD	Cephalic, cephalo-	SKIN	Derma, Integumentum
HEART	Cardium, cardiac, cardio-	STOMACH	Gastric, gastro-
INTESTINES	Cecum, colon, duode-num, ileum and jeju-num	TESTICLE	Orchio-, orchi-, orchido-
		URINARY BLADDER	Cysti-, cysto-
KIDNEY	Renal, nephric, nephro-	UTERUS	Hystero, metra
LIP	Cheil-	VAGINA	Vulvo, vaginal

PROOFREADER'S MARKS USED IN MANUSCRIPT TYPING

x	Change bad letter	#	Insert space	V	Equalize spacing
⌐	Raise	;/	Semicolon	:)	Colon
↓	Superior figure	⊙	Period	□	Em quad space
w.f.	Wrong font	⌐ or ⌐	Move to right	s.m.cap.	Small caps
	Push down space	tr.	Transpose	v	Less space
⌣	Lower	∧	Left out	◡	Close up
↑	Inferior figure	,	Insert comma	'	Apostrophe
. . .	Let it stand	Out, s.c.	Out, see copy	"	Quotation
stet /	Let it stand	Cap.	Capital letter	¶	Paragraph
9	Turn over	1/m	One-em dash	no.¶	No paragraph
≡	Straighten lines	ital.	Italics	b.f.	Bold face
⌐ or ⌐	Move to left	⅋ or ⅋	take out (dele)	=	Hyphen

MANUSCRIPT AND ABSTRACT
STYLE SHEET

While various journals each have a special style of their own and often submit a "style sheet" of instructions, either printed in the journal in question or included with returned galley proof, certain general rules are in order. Furthermore, much typing that the secretary does will not be for publication. The following is a selected list of general rules pertaining to style.

ABBREVIATIONS

cycles/sec   cycles per second
g   gram
kg   kilogram
m   meter
M   molar
mc   millicurie
mEq   milliequivalent
mg   milligram
ml   milliliter
mu   millimicron
msec   millisecond
μ micron
$\mu\mu$ micromicron
μc   microcurie
μg   microgram
μsec   microsecond
%   per cent
qO$_2$ oxygen consumed

GENERAL RULES

22 C (No degree sign)
Change auricle to atrium, auricles to atria
Change adrenalin to epinephrine
Capital X in X-ray
Change mercury to Hg (no period)
Write out "second" and "minute" except with
   use of diagonals; e.g., 1 ml/min

in vivo, in vitro, in situ, i.e., et al. are *not* to
   be underlined for italics
type II, group III, no. 3 (lower case "t", "g"
   and "n"

HYPHENATION

bundle-branch block
threefold (no hyphen)
end-diastolic
T 1824 (no hyphen)
P wave, S wave, Q wave (no hyphen)
2-year-old child
left-to-right shunt
l-norepinephrine
No hyphen after "non," "post" or "pre"
   (noninfectious, postoperative, preoperative)

NUMBERS

Use words through the number ten, except with abbreviations, units of measurement, in a series of numbers, and before %. Use numerals for larger numbers, beginning with 11.

In headings, spell out numerals below 100.

Ordinal numbers are to be spelled out (the eighth patient; on the tenth day).

Fractions to be written out, unless used with numeral (one-tenth, 6½).

SPELLINGS

Use long spelling (technique, not technic; physiological, not physiologic).

When there is a choice between "L" and "ll" in words such as pedaling (pedalling) and traveler (traveller), use only one "l".

(courtesy of: George E. Wakerlin, M.D., Ph.D.
American Heart Association, Inc.)

II

THE BODY AS A WHOLE

. . . For I am Fearfully and Wonderfully made. PSALM 139, 14

One must know the structure of the body in order to understand its functions. While the succeeding chapters are divided into systems and arranged by systems, (i.e., cardiovascular, muscular, etc.) these structures are interrelated and all work together to maintain the activity of the body as a whole.

The cell is the structural unit of the body. The body as a whole is an aggregation of cells. Therefore, it is best understood by dividing the body into systems and explaining here briefly the organs, tissues, unit patterns and cells.

SYSTEMS OF THE BODY

A system is an arbitrary arrangement of the organs of the body closely allied to one another and concerned with the same or related functions.

INTEGUMENTARY SYSTEM (SKIN)

The integumentary system consists of the skin, or integumentum, which covers the entire surface of the body, approximately 16 to 20 square feet in extent, continuous with that of the external orifices of the digestive, respiratory and urogenital systems. It holds a mirror to age and health and plays the diverse roles of raincoat, overcoat, sunshade, suit of armor and refrigerator. It is sensitive to touch, temperature and pain, and withstands the wear and tear of our lifetime while maintaining its own integrity.

SKELETAL SYSTEM

The skeletal system consists of the bones of the body which are held together by ligaments, and serves as the bony framework for the attachment of muscles. Its main functions are support, protection and the enablement of motion.

MUSCULAR SYSTEM

The muscular system consists of three types of muscles, striated muscle (skeletal muscle), the unstriated or smooth muscle (the muscle coats of the stomach and viscera) and indistinctly striated muscle (cardiac muscle). Their main function is to cause movement by contracting and relaxing. Skeletal muscles are usually attached to two or more bones.

NERVOUS SYSTEM

The nervous system is an intricate and complicated organization of structures concerned with the correlation and integration of bodily processes, the sensations and adjustments to its environment and with conscious life. This system is divided into three categories, namely, the Central Nervous System, the Peripheral Nervous System and the Autonomic Nervous System, all arbitrary and artificial but concerned with their essential unity in structure and their interdependence in function.

CARDIOVASCULAR SYSTEM

The cardiovascular system consists of the heart, the arteries, veins and capillaries. Its function is to distribute blood to all parts of the body and return it to the heart.

LYMPHATIC SYSTEM

The lymphatic system consists of lymphatic capillaries, the lymphatic vessels and the lymph nodes or glands. The function of the lymphatics is to carry lymph from all tissues to the veins. Lymphatics of the small intestine are called lacteals whose function is the absorption of digested food.

RESPIRATORY SYSTEM

The respiratory system consists of the nose, pharynx, larynx, trachea, bronchi and lungs. Its function is to provide oxygen to the body tissue and to rid it of excess carbon dioxide.

DIGESTIVE SYSTEM

The digestive system consists of the mouth, pharynx, esophagus, stomach, the small intestine (which is divided into the duodenum, jejunum and ileum), the large intestine (which is divided into the cecum, the colon, which itself is divided into the ascending colon, transverse colon, descending colon and sigmoid colon, the rectum and the anal canal. Accessory glands are the salivary glands (the parotid, submaxillary and sublingual), the pancreas, the liver and the gallbladder. The function of the digestive system is to receive, digest and absorb food and water and to eliminate waste products.

GENITOURINARY SYSTEM

The genitourinary system consists of the urinary organs, i.e., the kidneys, ureters, bladder and urethra for the secretion, storage and elimination of urine, and the genital organs, which are concerned with the process of reproduction.

MALE

The reproductive system in the male consists of two testicles, two epididymides, two vasa deferentia (ductus deferens), prostate, seminal vesicles, and ejaculatory ducts, penis and scrotum.

FEMALE

The reproductive system in the female consists of the ovaries, uterus, vagina and external genitalia, vagina, vulva and clitoris.

ENDOCRINE SYSTEM

The endocrine system, or system of ductless glands, includes the hypophysis or pituitary body, thyroid, parathyroids, thymus, suprarenal glands and portions of the glands with ducts, such as the islands of Langerhans in the pancreas, part of the ovaries and testes and parts of the liver, gastric and intestinal mucosa. The secretions of the endocrine or ductless glands are taken up directly by the blood stream and therefore are called the glands of internal secretion. The endocrine glands share with the nervous system in the control of all the activities of the body tissues; however, more frequently they control the slower changes, or adaptations of the body to its environment.

SENSORY SYSTEM

The sensory system is a subdivision of the central nervous system and consists of the organs of special sense which comprise hearing and equilibrium, vision, smell and taste, namely, the ears, eyes, nose and organ of taste, the taste-bud, most numerous upon the superior surface of the tongue.

ORGANS, TISSUES, UNIT PATTERNS AND CELLS

ORGANS

An organ is a member of a system, composed of a combination of tissues which together perform some specialized function not possible by separate tissues, and for which it is especially adapted.

Systems are composed of organs which act together to perform highly complex but specialized functions. An example of a system is the urinary system which consists of the following organs: (1) two kidneys, which secrete the urine by filtering waste materials from the blood; (2) two ureters, ducts which convey the urine from the kidneys to the bladder; (3) the bladder, a reservoir for the reception of urine; and (4) the urethra, a tube through which the urine passes from the bladder to the exterior of the body.

TISSUES

A tissue may be defined as an organization of like cells performing a special bodily function, bound together with an intercellular substance and bathed by extracellular fluid. The organs can be analyzed into component tissues. For example, the stomach is composed of columnar epithelial tissue, smooth muscle tissue, connective tissue and serous tissue.

1. *Connective tissue* forms the supporting framework of the body, and protects and binds together the other systems of the body.

2. *Muscular tissue* is specialized for the performance of work by its ability to contract and relax.

3. *Nervous tissue*, because of its specialized properties of irritability and conductivity, may carry impulses to all parts of the body, thus coordinating its functions.

UNIT PATTERN

A unit pattern, or functional unit, can be defined approximately as the smallest aggregate of cells which, when repeated many times, composes an organ. (Plates 1 and 2). These unit patterns are simple, minute and repeated a vast number of times to form the lobules (smallest macroscopic units), are composed of chains of cells with their definite supply paths of blood, lymph and nerve fibers

Some of the tissue arrangements stand out clearly on microscopic examinations because the pattern which they make is unique; receiving names such as alveolus or pulmonary unit, nephron of kidney (renal tubule), chain of cells of the liver, reflex arc of the nervous system and Haversian system of bone. These units, both structural and physiological, are referred to as a unit pattern or functional unit.

CELLS

Cells are the physiological and structural units of the body. Low down in the scale of life are simple animals consisting of one cell. These unicellular animals carry on the biological functions which are essential to life. These biological functions are breathing, digesting, collecting and distributing, excreting, response to environment and reproduction. The amoeba, a typical one-celled organism, can be observed under the microscope carrying on all of these functions. The life of each individual cell in the body is dependent on its ability to carry on these biological functions.

Higher in the scale of life are animals that consist of a greater number of cells. Man may be described as a multicellular animal consisting of an enormous number of cells and intercellular material which the cells have made. In multicellular animals, individual cells are often remote from air, food and the excreting organs and must rely upon the circulating fluids to carry oxygen and food to them and waste matters from them. The systems of the body represent an adaptation and specialization of groups of cells to carry on the biological activities for the body as a whole.

A comparison of the biological activities of a unicellular animal with the biological activities of the cells of multicellular animals and the functions performed by the systems of the body shows them to be essentially the same.

STRUCTURE OF THE CELL

A cell is a minute portion of living substance edged by a cell membrane, thin and delicate, as shown in Plate 3.

Man belongs to the group of animals known as vertebrates, characterized by possession of a back bone or vertebral column. In describing the body it is assumed that, in the case of man, he is in the anatomic position—standing erect, the arms at the sides and the palms turned forward (Plates 4 & 5; Table 1).

The cavities of the body consist of:

1. Dorsal cavity, (Plate 5) which contains the brain and spinal cord, is divided into the cranial cavity formed by the bones of the skull, and the vertebral cavity, formed by the vertebrae.

2. Ventral cavity (Plate 5), which is divided into the thoracic and abdominopelvic cavities. (1) The thoracic cavity is subdivided into right and left pleural cavities, which contain the lungs, the pericardial cavity, which contains the heart, and the mediastinum, which contains the trachea, bronchi, esophagus and thymus gland; blood and lymph vessels lie between these subdivisions in the thoracic cavity. (2) The abdominopelvic cavity has two portions which are continuous, in an upper abdominal part and a lower pelvic

portion. (a) The abdominal portion contains the liver, gallbladder, stomach, spleen, pancreas and small and large intestines. (b) The pelvic portion contains the bladder, rectum and sigmoid colon. In the female, the pelvic portion has in addition, two ovaries, uterine tubes and uterus; in the male, the prostate gland, seminal vesicles and a part of the ductus deferens. The organs contained in any of the three great body cavities are called viscera.

All of these systems are closely interrelated and dependent on each other. While each forms a unit especially adapted for the performance of some function, that function cannot be performed without the cooperative activity of the other systems. It is the function of the body fluids, and the nervous system to integrate the work of the systems.

TABLE I

Anatomical positions

Terms	Name	Explanation	Terms	Name	Explanation
Plane or section	Sagittal	Vertical plane or section dividing body into right and left portions.	Relative position or direction	Cranial (cranoid) or cephalic (Cephalad)	Nearest or toward head
	Midsagittal	Vertical at midline; dividing body into right and left halves		Caudal (Caudad)	Away from head
	Frontal or coronal	Vertical, but at right angles to sagittal sections, dividing body into anterior (front) and posterior (back) portions		Medial (Mesad)	Middle or nearest midsagittal plane
				Lateral (laterally)	Side or farthest from midsagittal plane
	Transverse	Horizontal, hence at right angles to both sagittal and frontal sections, dividing body into upper and lower portions		Proximal (Proximally)	Near source or attachment
				Distal (Distally)	Away from source or attachment
Surface or relative position	Anterior or ventral	Front of body, hence on or nearest abdominal surface		Afferent	In relation to nerves or blood vessels-conducting toward structure or organ
	Posterior or dorsal	Back of body			
	Superior or inferior	Upper or higher Lower		Efferent	Conducting away from structure or organ

III

ANATOMIC SYSTEMS OF THE BODY

SKELETAL SYSTEM

. . .That God made man upright. . . ECCLESIASTES 7, 29.

. . .And the bones came together, bone to its bone, . . .and . . .lo, there were sinews upon them, and the flesh came up, and skin covered them . . .
EZEKIEL 37, 7 & 8

The skeleton forms the bony framework on which the soft tissue of the body is supported and serves as the basis of attachment for muscles, thus maintaining their definite position in the body. The skeleton affords a strong system of levers, by means of which the muscles may change the position of the body as a whole or of its various parts. To serve such functions the skeleton must be strong, elastic, must permit movement without undue effort, yet also without any serious lessening of its strength. These ends are accomplished by stout and hard yet somewhat elastic material (bone) and (cartilage), and by connecting these bones by means of joints (articulations) at which the firm structures can move upon one another without significant resistance and yet securely, because they are appropriately attached to each other.

Bones may be considered as organs because they are made up of osseous tissue, cartilage, fibrous tissue, nervous tissue and vascular tissue, and because they function as integral parts of the skeletal system.

CARTILAGES

The embryonic skeleton is formed of fibrous membranes and hyaline cartilage, beginning in these two tissues in the eighth week of embryonic life. Bone formed in a membrane is known as intramembranous bone; bone formed in cartilage is known as endochondral bone, and indicates only the method by which the development of bone begins. Tissue termed bone is thus formed from mesenchyme by the cementing substance of differentiating connective tissue condensing between the fibrils and enclosing cells to form an osteoid tissue which later calcifies.

Cartilage is dense connective tissue consisting of cells embedded in ground substance or matrix, and of a white or gray color, semiopaque and is avascular. Cartilage is tough, yet elastic and compressible. In the adult skeleton, cartilage completes a part of the skeleton in the thorax (costal cartilages of the ribs), the nasal septum, in the external ear and in the trachea and bronchi. Cartilage lines the Eustachian tube and the wall of the larynx. Cartilage holds bones firmly together as in the vertebral column, and fills up intervals between bones, as in certain parts of the skull; it covers the articular surfaces of bones. Articular cartilage discs, or menisci, are partial or complete fibrocartilage plates interposed between two articular surfaces (interarticular cartilages).

ARTICULATIONS

Articulations are the connection of bones and can, as a whole, be divided into synar-

31

throdial or immovable joints and diarthrodial or movable joints. Diarthroidal joints possess a synovial cavity permitting easy movement, and this cavity may be wholly or partly divided by an interarticular cartilage or meniscus into two parts. The synovial cavity contains a joint lubricating fluid called synovia. Synarthrodial joints are firmly fixed by interlocking of the bones concerned or by interposition of a thick but strong layer of fibrocartilage over a large area on each of the bones.

LIGAMENTS

Ligaments are bands of flexible connective tissue which pass over a joint connecting the articular ends of bones. They are best developed over diarthrodial joints, where the articulating bones have no connecting medium between them. If the ligaments are not to be a hindrance to free movement, they must be so arranged with regard to the joint surfaces, and be so shaped with reference to the ligamentous attachments that any given ligament will either be tense and effective at one part of the movement or will remain tense, and tense throughout it. Ligaments then consist of fibrous material, folds of thickened peritoneum and the remains of fetal structures.

BONES

Bones constitute the larger part of the skeleton. Bone is extremely hard, but at the same time exhibits a small amount of elasticity and toughness. It is composed of animal or organic matter impregnated with earthy salts; about one-third or less of animal matter and the rest as mineral matter. The former gives toughness and the latter hardness to bone.

Bone exists in two states in the body, according to its presentation: compact (found on the exterior of all bones), and cancellus (spongy tissue simulating latticework found in the interior).

The skeleton comprises the axial skeleton and those forming the appendicular skeleton. The former makes up the skull, vertebral column and thorax; the latter consists of the bones of the upper and lower extremities (Plates 6-9). The various bones are divided, according to their shape and appearance into short, long, flat and irregular bones. Depressions in bone may be described as follows:

(1) Fossa—a pit or hollow.
(2) Groove—a furrow.
(3) Sulcus—a cavity within a bone, also designates grooves on the inner surface of the skull.
(4) Foramen canal—a hole or opening in a bone.
(5) Meatus—a tubelike passageway.

Therefore, depressions on the surfaces of bones may be fossae, cavities, fossettes, or foveae; if more linear (measure of length) in direction, grooves or sulci; if a large cavity exists in a bone it may be described as a sinus, cell or antrum.

Prominences of bone varying from the general level are projections described as follows:

(1) Processes, a general term for any bony prominence.
(2) Spine or spinous processes—a sharp projection.
(3) Tubercle—a small rounded projection.
(4) Tuberosity—a large rounded projection.
(5) Crest—a prominent ridge.
(6) Condyle—a protruded mass carrying an articular surface.
(7) Head—an enlargement at the end of a bone beyond the constricted portion, or neck.
(8) Trochanters—(runner) either of two processes below the neck of the femur.

And, if more linear in disposition, they are referred to as ridges, spines, crests or lines.

A projecting articular process on a bone is frequently referred to as the head, its narrowed attachment to the rest of the bone as the neck, and the remainder constitutes the body, or in a long bone, the shaft. A condyle is a rounded protuberance at the end of a bone forming an articulation, and a ramus is a broad arm or process of bone projecting from the main body (a branch of one of the divisions of a forked structure).

The bones are preformed in the embryo as condensations of mesenchyme, which in most cases becomes cartilagenous before ossification begins; but some are unchondrified, that is they do not convert to cartilage. As stated earlier in this chapter, the bones are formed in cartilage and fibrous membrane. These terms imply that the bones have replaced cartilage or noncartilagenous "membrane."

The process of ossification is essentially similar in both varieties of formation, except that in chondral ossification the cartilage is calcified first and then absorbed and replaced by the true bony formation. Certain large cells called osteoblasts have the power of depositing or forming bone around themselves; they exist in the covering tissues of the developing bone, periosteum and perichondrium, and in the case of chondral ossification they grow into the cartilage and occupy the spaces made in that structure by the confluence (running together) of the cell spaces which goes with calcification. The early bone thus formed is removed by the action of other cells known as osteoclasts, and in this way a medullary cavity is provided in long bones while additional bone is being laid down on the surface under the periosteum, so that the bone increases in thickness.

The greater part of the skeleton is composed of cartilage bones, including that of the limbs, trunk and base of skull; the bones of the face and vault of the skull are formed in membrane. The chondral (cartilage) skeleton is the modified endoskeleton or internal bony framework of the body, and constitutes a part of the skeleton occurring in the costal cartilages of the ribs, nasal septum, in the external ear and lining the Eustachian tube, in the wall of the larynx, in the trachea and bronchi, between bodies of the vertebrae and covering the articular surfaces of bones. It forms the major portion of the embryonic skeleton. The bony framework of the body consists of 206 bones.

AXIAL SKELETON

SKULL

The skull can be divided for descriptive purposes into a facial and a cranial part. The cranial bones form the walls of the cavity that contains the brain and the face bones are situated below the front portion of this "brain box." The skull is composed of 22 bones, which, with the exception of the lower jaw, are immovably articulated (joined) with each other. The hyoid is the U-shaped bone situated in the ventral floor of the pharynx below the base of the tongue and in front of the epiglottis.

VERTEBRAL COLUMN

The human spinal column is made up of 33 bones or vertebrae, as a part of the axial skeleton. The length of the column of bones is much increased by intervertebral discs, of fibrocartilage placed between the segments, which add greatly to the elasticity of the column. The column has two main functions: (1) support of the trunk and transmission of its weight to the pelvis and lower extremities; (2) protection of the spinal cord and its membranes.

The vertebral column is divided into five regions in which vertebrae show characteristic modifications, such as thoracic region, cervical region, etc. Above this, in the neck and supporting the skull, are seven cervical vertebrae, and between the thorax and pelvis are five lumbar segments. The thoracic vertebrae are 12 in number, and carry the movable ribs. Below this are the five sacral vertebrae, fused together to form the sacrum and firmly fixed between the bony side walls of the pelvis, and the sacrum rapidly tapers below to give place to the degenerated coccyx, usually four in number and called "false vertebrae"; the presacral segments are termed the "true vertebrae."

THORAX

The thoracic skeleton is attached dorsally to the vertebral column. It contains a series of 12 ribs on each side, connected with a central sternum in front by a means of costal cartilages. Of each series of 12 ribs, only the upper seven have their cartilages directly connected with the sternum; the next three cartilages join the one immediately above, so only reach the sternum indirectly, and the two last ribs have their short cartilagenous ends terminating without such junction, lying in the muscles of the body wall.

The upper seven pairs are termed true or sternal ribs; the remainder are false or asternal, the last two ribs on each side are referred to as "floating ribs." There are some-times eight sternal ribs.

The wall of the thorax is completed by intercostal muscles and membranes in the intercostal spaces between the ribs, and pleura (serous membrane) lines it on its inner side.

The ribs and sternum constitute a firm but movable thoracic cage protecting the viscera (internal organs, especially the abdominal viscera). The firmness due to the bony elements prevents collapse from atmospheric pressure, the lungs being expanded. The power of movement is associated, of course, with respiration.

The sternum is a long flat bone which lies in the front wall of the chest, having the true costal cartilages attached to its sides.

APPENDICULAR SKELETON

The term "limb" is applied to one of the appendages (an arm or a leg) which are freely movable on the "body" and distinct from it, bearing in mind that these are only what one may call free, and are carried by a more fixed part related to them and embedded in the walls of the trunk. These embedded parts, really applied to the surface of the proper body wall, constitute the pectoral and pelvic girdles: in the former, the skeleton is capable of movement and not firmly articulated with the trunk skeleton; but in the latter, where stability and strength are necessary for carrying the weight of the body, the girdle is firmly fixed to the sacrum and forms with it the bony pelvis.

The *pectoral* girdle consists of the scapula and clavicle on each side: the clavicle is the only bony connection between the scapula and the trunk skeleton articulating (being jointed) with the sternum. The upper arm, the proximal segment of the free limb, has the humerus as its bony skeleton, articulating with the scapula and carrying the bones of the forearm (radius and ulna) at its distal end.

The *pelvic* girdle is formed by two hip bones, which articulate with each other ventrally and with the sacrum dorsally. Each of these is composed of three bones joined together, the ilium, ischium and pubis, and has a deep articular surface (acetabulum) which carries the femur that supports the thigh. The ilium is on the dorsal and upper side of the acetabulum, the ischium and pubis on its ventral side, and the junction of one hip bone with the other is effected by the meeting of their pubic portions in the symphysis. All the three parts of the bone are concerned in forming the acetabulum.

SURGICAL PROCEDURES— SKELETAL SYSTEM

Bones

Incision

Aspiration biopsy of bone marrow, including sternal puncture.

Incision of soft tissue abscess.

Removal of metal band, plate, screw or nail.

Osteotomy: cutting, division or transection of bone, with or without internal fixation, pertaining to the clavicle, humerus, radius (malunited Colles' fracture), femur, subtrochanteric, femur supracondylar, tibia, lesser bones, correction of bowlegs or knock-knees.

Excision

Sequestrectomy: The surgical removal of sequestra, a piece of dead bone which has become separated during the process of necrosis from the sound bone.

Biopsy bone, may be superficial or deep.

Claviculectomy: may be either partial or total.

Astragalectomy: Excision of the astragalus (ball of the ankle joint).

Excision of head of radius.

Carpectomy: surgical excision of one or more of the carpal bones.

Coccygectomy: excision of the coccyx.

Claviculectomy: cutting or dividing the clavicle.

Coccygotomy: surgical removal of the coccyx.

Patellectomy: excision or removal of the patella.

Hemipelvectomy: amputation of a lower limb through the sacroiliac joint.

Metatarsectomy: surgical excision or resection of the metatarsus.

Excision of bone marrow.

Excision of bone cyst, chrondroma or

exostosis, in either large or small bones.

Costectomy: excising or resecting a rib.

Craterization, buttering or saucerization of bone.

Diaphysectomy: removal of part of the shaft of a long bone in either the femur, tibia, humerus, radius or fibula.

Radical resection of bone for tumor and including bone graft in either a major or a minor bone.

Hemiphalangectomy: excision of part of a digital phalanx for hallux valgus.

Introduction

Insertion of wire (Kirschner wire).

Insertion of metal pin (Steinmann pin).

Insertion of caliper or tongs.

Insertion of threaded or beaded wire.

Repair

Osteoplasty: The plastic repair of bones or shortening of bone, such as the femur, tibia, humerus, radius, ulna or other bones. Mandibular repair for prognathism or micrognathism.

Bone Graft

Osteoperiosteal graft; periosteal graft, and including obtaining and placing graft.

Bone graft: Femur, tibia, humerus, radius, ulna.

Autogenous, originating within the body, i.e., grafted to face or skull and including taking and placing graft.

Cartilage graft, autogenous, originating within the body, i.e., grafting to face or skull and including taking and placing graft.

Bone or cartilage graft: (a) Homograft; isograft: taken from another person; (b) Autograft: taken from another part of the same individual; (c) Heterograft: having a different or dissimilar origin, e.g. taken from an animal.

Spinal fusion: with partial excision of intervertebral disc. May be of more than two segments.

Lumbosacral fusion

Scapulopexy: Surgical fixation of the scapula to the ribs.

Patellapexy: Suturing the patella to the lower end of the femur.

Pectus thorax: excavatum—infants—plastic repair; congenital deformity of thorax with sternum depressed.

Pectus excavatum (major) plastic repair.

Epiphyseal: diaphyseal fusion; epiphyseal arrest; epiphysiodesis, femur, tibia and fibula combined (femur, tibia and fibula) combined (upper and lower tibial and fibular).

Freeing of bone adhesions, callus, or synostosis.

Fractures

Manipulation

Skull, nonoperative, also depressed with operation.

Facial Bones

Nasal, simple, closed reduction; compound, closed reduction; simple or compound, open reduction.

Malar, simple closed reduction; simple or compound, depressed, open reduction; and may include multiple surgical approaches.

Maxilla, simple, closed reduction; simple or compound, closed reduction; and may include wiring of teeth.

Other fractures of maxilla include simple, multiple, or compound; complicated; open reduction; and fixation by traction, head caps, multiple internal fixation, etc.

Mandible, simple, closed reduction; simple or compound, closed reduction and including of teeth; open reduction; skeletal pinning with external fixation.

Spine and Trunk

Vertebral body, closed reduction, one or more than one.

Sacrum, compound, simple, or with operation.

Clavicle, simple, closed reduction; simple or compound, open reduction.

Scapula, simple, closed reduction, plus acromial process; simple, closed reduction; simple or compound, open reduction.

Sternum, simple, nondepressed, closed reduction; or compound.

Ribs, simple strapping, complicated.

Pelvis (Ilium, Ischim, Pubis)

Fracture, simple, closed reduction; complicated, closed reduction; one or more bones, simple or compound, open reduction.

Acetabulum, with or without other fractures of pelvis, simple, closed reduction, no displacement; central, with displacement; simple or compound, open reduction.

Upper Extremity

Humerus, surgical neck, simple, either not requiring manipulation or requiring manipulation with general anesthesia. Simple or compound, open reduction.

Shaft, simple, closed reduction: Simple, closed, reduction with general anesthesia, simple or compound, open reduction.

Elbow (distal end of humerus, proximal end of radius, proximal end of ulna), condyle only, simple closed reduction, simple or compound open reduction.

Skeletal pinning with external fixation supracondylar, olecranon, open reduction.

Radius, head, simple, closed reduction head, simple or compound, open reduction; shaft, simple, closed reduction, without displacement.
simple, closed reduction with displacement.
simple or compound, open reduction.

Distal end, Colles' (including ulnar styloid) simple, closed reduction; simple or compound, open reduction. Skeletal pinning with external fixation.

Ulna, shaft, simple, closed reduction and may be with displacement and with general anesthesia. Simple or compound, open reduction. Skeletal pinning with external fixation.

Radius and ulna, simple closed reduction and may be with general anesthesia; simple or compound, open reduction. Skeletal pinning with external fixation.

Carpal bones, one, simple, closed reduction; simple or compound, open reduction.

Metacarpal, one, simple, closed reduction; one, simple or compound, open reduction. Skeletal pinning with external fixation.

Phalanx or phalanges, one finger, or thumb, simple, closed reduction; one finger, or thumb, compound; simple or compound, open reduction.

Lower Extremity

Femur, neck, simple, closed reduction, with fixation; neck, simple or compound, open reduction; multiple pinning, and with or without external fixation.

Intertrochanteric, simple, closed reduction with fixation; simple, open reduction.

Slipped epiphysis, closed reduction with fixation; open reduction, acute; reconstructive, including supracondylar, simple, or closed reduction.

Femur, compound with general anesthesia; simple or compound, open reduction.

Skeletal pinning with external fixation.

Knee (distal end of femur, proximal end of tibia, proximal end of fibula), femur or tibia, condyle-closed reduction, compound with general anesthesia; simple or compound, open reduction, two condyles.

Patella, simple or compound with general anesthesia; simple, open reduction.

Tibia, shaft, simple, closed reduction with general anesthesia;
simple or compound, open reduction.

Malleolus, simple, closed reduction;
simple or compound, open reduction;

Fibula, shaft, simple, closed reduction;
simple or compound, open reduction.

Malleolus, simple, closed reduction,
simple or compound, open reduction.

Tibia and Fibula, shafts, simple, closed reduction; compound with general anesthesia;
simple or compound, open reduction.

Skeletal pinning with external fixation.

Ankle, bimalleolar (including Potts) simple, closed reduction;
compound with general anesthesia;
simple or compound, open reduction.

Trimalleolar, simple, closed reduction; compound, with general anesthesia; or simple or compound, open reduction.

Tarsal (except astragalus and os calcis), one, simple, closed reduction
one, compound with general anesthesia;
one, simple or compound, open reduction.

Astragalus: Simple, closed reduction; compound, with general anesthesia; or simple or compound, open reduction.

Os Calcis; simple, closed reduction; compound, with general anesthesia; or simple or compound, open reduction. Skeletal pinning with external fixation

Metatarsal, simple, closed reduction; one, compound, with general anesthesia;
one, simple or compound, open reduction.

Phalanx or phalanges, one toe, simple, closed reduction; or one toe, simple or compound, open reduction.

Joints

Incision

Arthrotomy or capsulotomy with exploration, drainage or removal of loose body, e.g., osteochondritis or foreign body, in the shoulder, elbow, wrist, other joints of upper extremity, hip, knee, ankle, other joints of lower extremity, finger, one, toe, one.

Arthrocentesis: puncture for aspiration of joint, or injection of medication.

Sesamoid bone, excision, one or more.

Excision

Arthrectomy: excision of joint; punch biopsy of synovial membrane; temporomandibular joint; excision of intervertebral disc with spinal fusion.

Excision of neural arch and nerve exploration for spondylolisthesis.

Meniscectomy: excision of semilunar cartilage of knee joint.

Menisectomy of temporomandibular joint.

Synovectomy: excision of synovial membrane of any one of the following; elbow, hip, knee, ankle.

Introduction

Arthrography: injection of air or radiopaque material into joint for roentgenographic examination.

Repair

Arthroplasty: plastic or reconstructive operation on any joint, any type, e.g., shoulder, elbow, wrist, finger, one joint; hip, knee, ankle, toe, one joint; metatarsophalangeal joint; bunion operation.

Arthrodesis: fusion of joint, with or without tendon transplant, as in the following: shoulder, elbow, wrist, finger, thumb, one joint; hip, knee, ankle, hammer toes, operation, one toe; hallux rigidus, repair of; tarsal, joints, one or more; other joints, lower extremity; foot, triple arthrodesis, unilateral; foot, with tendon transplantation; stabilization of joints by bone block.

Suture

Capsulorrhaphy: suture or repair of joint capsule for recurrent dislocation of shoulder or patella.

Suture of torn, ruptured or severed collateral ligaments of the knee.

Suture of torn, ruptured or severed cruciate ligaments of the knee.

Reconstruction, both collateral or cruciate ligaments of the knee.

Reconstruction both collateral ligaments of the ankle.

Reconstruction both metacarpophalangeal or interphalangeal ligaments.

Manipulation

Manipulation of joint under anesthesia, including application of cast, or traction. Includes shoulder, elbow, wrist, digits, one or more, under anesthesia where no other surgical procedure is performed; hip, knee, ankle, spine.

Manipulation of shoulder for fibrous ankylosis, under general anesthesia.

Turnbuckle jacket, body only, for scoliosis.

Turnbuckle spica jacket for scoliosis.

Club foot and application of cast, also an edging cast.

Dislocations

Temporomandibular: simple, closed reduction.

Vertebra, cervical, simple, closed reduction, with anesthesia; cervical, simple or compound, with operation; dorsal, simple or compound with operation.

Dorsal, simple, closed reduction with general anesthesia.

Lumbar, simple, closed reduction with general anesthesia.

Lumbar, simple or compound, with operation.

Clavicle, sternoclavicular: simple, closed reduction; compound, with general anesthesia; simple or compound, open reduction; acromioclavicular, simple, closed reduction; simple or compound, open reduction.

Shoulder (humerus), simple, closed reduction; simple or compound, open reduction.

Elbow, simple, closed reduction; compound, with general anesthesia; or simple or compound, open reduction.

Wrist, carpal, one bone, simple, closed reduction; compound, with general anesthesia; or simple or compound, open reduction.

Metacarpal, one bone, simple, closed reduction; one bone, simple or compound, open reduction.

Finger, one, one or more joints, simple or compound, closed reduction; simple or compound, open reduction.

Thumb, simple or compound, closed reduction; simple or compound, open reduction.

Thumb, simple or compound, closed reduction; simple or compound, open reduction.

Hip (femur), simple, closed reduction; simple or compound, open reduction; congenital, closed reduction.

Knee (tibia), simple; closed reduction; compound, with general anesthesia; or simple or compound, open reduction.

Patella, simple, closed reduction; compound, with general anesthesia; or simple or compound, open reduction.

Ankle, simple, closed reduction; compound, with general anesthesia; or simple or compound, open reduction.

Tarsal, simple, closed reduction; compound, with general anesthesia; or simple or compound, open reduction.

Astragalo-tarsal, simple, closed reduction; compound, with general anesthesia; or simple or compound, open reduction.

Metatarsal, one bone, simple or compound, closed reduction.

Toe, one, simple or compound, closed reduction; simple or compound, open reduction; one or more joints, simple or compound, closed reduction.

Bursae

Incision

Drainage infected bursa.

Removal of subdeltoid calcereous deposits.

Removal of subtrochanteric calcereous deposits.

Puncture for aspiration of bursae

Needling of bursa, with irrigation of bursa.

Excision

Radical excision of bursae, forearm, viz., tenosynovitis fungosa, Tbs. and other granulomas.

Excision of bursa, olecranon, prepatellar, subacromial and ischial.

Cineplastic Procedures

Amputation of an extremity in which muscles and tendons are so arranged in the stump that they will execute independent movements and communicate motion to specially constructed prosthetic apparatuses.

Amputation: Upper Extremity

Interthoracoscapular.

Disarticulation of shoulder.

Arm through humerus.

Forearm, through radius and ulna.

Guillotine upper arm with subsequent revision or reamputation.

Scapulothoracic.

Disarticulation of wrist.

Hand through metacarpal bones.

Metacarpal, with finger or thumb, one with split or Wolff graft; or skinplasty or tenodesis, with definitive resection or tenodesis, with definitive resection volar digital nerves.

Amputation: Lower Extremity

Interpelviabdominal

Disarticulation of hip.

Disarticulation of knee.

Thigh through femur, including supra-condylar.

Guillotine, thigh with subsequent revision or reamputation.

Leg, through tibia and fibula.

Guillotine, leg, with subsequent revision or reamputation.

Ankle (Syme, Pirogoff), with skinplasty and resection of nerves.

Foot, transmetatarsal, or midtarsal each foot.

Metatarsal with toe, split or Wolff graft, or skin plasty or tenodesis, with

definitive resection of digital nerves.

Toe, any joint or phalanx.

Toe, more than one, split or Wolff graft, or skin plasty or tenodesis, with definitive resection of digital nerves.

Repair

Freeing of web fingers, with flaps, or with graft.

Plaster Casts

Molded plaster cast include: to fore-arm; elbow to fingers; hand and wrist; shoulder to hand; shoulder spica; ankle (foot to mid leg), or knee (foot to thigh); ambulatory leg cast; molded plaster to leg; spica, unilateral (hip to foot), bilateral; body, shoulder to hips, including head; wedging cast.

INTEGUMENTARY SYSTEM

Thou hast clothed me with skin and flesh. JOB 10, 11

Integumentum (skin) covers the entire surface of the body and its epithelium. The epithelium is also a cellular, avascular layer covering all the free surfaces, cutaneous, mucous and serous, including the glands and other structures derived therefrom. Skin is continuous with that of the external orifices of the digestive, respiratory and urogenital systems. It is smooth in some areas, soft in others and hairy in still others. In some areas, skin is thick, horny and taut, but thin, translucent and pliable in others. Skin is firm over bony regions, may glide easily and may be relaxed or flabby. The amount and nature of the secretion of the cutaneous glands in any one region make skin rough, smooth, dry or moist.

The color of the skin differs greatly from individual to individual, determined by the difference in the amount of pigments, in vascularity and in the thickness of the dead outer layer.

Skin is the barrier as well as the principal organ of communication between man and his environment, and most of our contacts with the environment are through the skin. Since living cells must be surrounded with

lymph, the contact of the body with the air is made by means of dead cells, forming a protective covering for the living cells. Living cells of the inner layers of the skin are constantly pushed to the outside, shrinking and undergoing progressive chemical changes which cement them firmly together and render them waterproof, thus a tissue-fluid environment is maintained for living cells, although man lives in an air environment.

As an example of the importance of the skin's role in this tissue-fluid environment, if untreated, burns of one-third of the skin's area may be fatal due to fluid loss, involving as much as three quarters of the patient's plasma within the first few hours, the proportion of fluid to red cells falling so rapidly that the blood cannot function.

Skin reflects the well-being or the disorders of the organism. It is a turbulent tissue, and it grows, differentiates and renews itself at all times. Skin is versatile, performing numerous functions and producing several and different end products.

The skin has many functions such as covering the body and protecting the deeper tissues from drying and injury, and protecting from invasion by infectious organisms. In many ways it is important in temperature regulation, by evaporation from its surface and by the regulations of the blood flow in the vessels. It has excretory functions, such as eliminating water with the various salts which compose perspiration. It has absorbing powers, and is an important light screen for underlying living cells.

Skin is stratified tissue. At the surface is the epithelium called epidermis, underlying this is a connective tissue layer, the dermis. A fatty layer, or panniculus adiposus, underlies the dermis. Beneath this fatty layer is a discontinuous, flat sheet of skeletal muscle, the panniculus carnosus; this layer separates the rest of the body tissues from the skin or integumentum. Widely distributed in the dermis are bundles of smooth muscle fibers, arrectores pilorum, attached to hair follicles. Smooth, oriented muscle fibers are found in the dermis of the scrotum and the penis, which form a relatively continuous layer called the tunica dartos. These fibers are also numerous in the nipple and areola of the breast, in the perineal (mass of tissue composed of skin, muscle and fascia) between the vagina and rectum in the female, the urethra and rectum of the male, and circumanal regions. The structure of the skin is shown in Plate 10.

The skin is held in place and attached to deeper structures by tela subcutanea tistues. Skin is bound to the deeper tissues over the palms, soles, joint flexures, scalp and auricles, but movable elsewhere.

Integumentary appendages such as hairs, nails and cutaneous glands, sebaceous glands and tactile buds grow directly from the epidermis and are integral parts of the skin. Skin is thinner on the ventral and flexor surfaces than it is on the dorsal and extensor surfaces. It is thicker in men than in women; however, in women, the tela subcutanea is usually thicker. The tela subcutanea is especially thick on the back, buttocks, thighs and upper leg region. The capacity of the skin to move and be stretched depends on its own thickness, the number of its folds, its intrinsic elasticity, firmness of fixation by the tela subcutanea and on the age of the individual. The skin of the abdomen

has the greatest capacity for distention. Tears called striae gravidarum appear as red streaks on the surface of the skin. After childbirth tears remain as permanent white lines called linae albicantes. Sudden increase of weight could cause similar lines on other parts of the body.

In infants skin is relatively free of creases. Skin, in addition to the wrinkles and furrows which are acquired with age and with use, possesses congenital flexure lines. These fixed creases, or "skin joints," indicate planes of firmer anchoring of the skin and the arrangement of collagenous fibers in the dermis.

Definite patterns of flexure lines, ridges, furrows and folds are formed in the embryo. They remain unchanged during the lifetime of each individual and can be altered only by damaging the underlying dermis. Dermatoglyphics is the study of the detail of these markings of the skin, especially those of the hands and feet.

The cleavage lines of Langer describe the specific pattern of grooves or furrows in the skin over the body. While roughly similar but certainly not identical in all individuals, they are oriented so as to represent the direction of elastic tension of the skin, at least in the cadaver. Recently it has been shown that the dynamic "wrinkle lines" of the living do not always agree with Langer's lines of the cadaver.

A peculiar topographic uniqueness in the skin of man is that the various regions of the face, scalp, the axilla and the abdomen are as different from each other as the skin of different species might be. Whereas hair follicles of the scalp of men in certain circumstances undergo regressive (receding) aging, changes in response to androgen (the male hormone), these hair follicles over the remainder of the body mostly grow larger under the same influence.

Skin disorders may be intrinsic, extrinsic and psychosomatic.

EPIDERMIS

Stratified squamous epithelium covers the entire surface of the body. Squamous cells are in the upper strata, flat and scale-like. Living cells are either cuboidal, columnar, fusiform or polyhedral. Dendritic melanocytes manufacture melanin granules, the skin pigment, and are scattered between the lower cells of the basal layers of the epidermis. The cells in the basal layer in human epidermis are usually cuboidal or columnar.

Epidermis is composed of a living stratum Malpighii, resting upon the dermis, and a dead, horny, superficial stratum corneum. Stratum Malpighii is subdivided into several layers. First, the one-celled deep basal layer, stratum basale or stratum germinativum, which is in contact with the dermis; above this is a layer of variable thicknesses, the stratum spinosum. These latter ascend to the surface, accumulate granules, and the cells together form a granular layer, stratum granulosum. A thin hyalin layer, just above the granular layer, is found in all human epidermis. The outer dead layer of the epidermis, stratum corneum, is composed of flattened cells resembling scales.

DERMIS

The epidermis and the cutaneous appendages, nails and hair, grow upon the dermis. The dermis is the deeper interlacing network of connective tissue fibers which constitute the major part of the total skin thickness. A superficial papillary layer or body and a deep reticular layer make up the dermis. One of the most characteristic features of the skin of man is a well-developed papillary body. This papillary body forms the connective tissue sheath around hair follicles, and the cutaneous appendages that extend into the dermis, pierce the reticular layer, and are accompanied by the papillary body throughout their length.

Collagenous fiber consists of a branching wavy band which is colorless and shows faint longitudinal striations. Reticular fiber branches and forms a network, and is found throughout connective tissue comprising about 38% of the entire weight of skin. Elastic fibers in the dermis are coarse, branching, cylindrical, or flat ribbons entwined among the collagenous tissues.

During development, the nerve net is the first ordered structure to appear in the dermis, and may influence the development of the cutaneous appendages. The plan of the dermal nerve networks varies with the density of the cutaneous appendages. In regions heavily populated with hair follicles, most of the cutaneous sensory nerves are distributed around them, but where follicles are sparse, the nerve networks are prominent. Smooth muscle, sebaceous glands, sweat glands and the thickness of the dermis itself all have a profound influence upon the particular form of the nerve networks.

HAIR OR PILARY SYSTEM

Hairs are dead keratinized cells that are compactly cemented together. Hair follicles grow out of tubes of epidermis, sunken into the dermis. Together with the sebaceous glands which grow from their sides, the dilated end or bulb which caps a dermal papilla, hair follicles form the pilosebaceous systems.

Hair follicles appear first at the end of the second and in the early part of the third fetal months, in the eyebrows, upper lip and chin. They appear slightly later on the forehead and scalp, and almost simultaneously. Hair follicle anlagen do not begin to appear on the trunk and appendages until the fourth and fifth fetal months. Development, therefore, begins on the head and spreads in a cephalocaudal progression.

Hair follicles are first to be formed from the relatively undifferentiated epidermis. This first sign of development is described as a crowding of cells at spaced focal spots in the basal layer of the epidermis, thus causing a slight bulging of the epidermis on its underside. Of many types, hairs may be long, short, stiff, soft, thin or thick, wooly, colored or white and spiny. The hair follicles are continuous with the surface epidermis by way of the pilary gland; slanted, their roots grow down to the panniculus adiposus and attain their greatest diameter at their base where they are dilated into an onion-shaped bulb. This bulb contains an obovate "cavity" which is completely filled with loose connective tissue of the dermal papilla. The pilary canal is the upper part of the hair follicle, extending from the entrance of the duct of the sebaceous glands to the surface. The arrectores pilorum muscles, (bundles of smooth muscle fibers), extend at an acute angle from the surface of the dermis to the bulge, a swelling on the side of the hair follicle, just below the level of the sebaceous glands. Innervated largely by adrenergic nerves, these muscles contract under stress, pull the hair to a vertical position and draw the skin around the follicles, causing elevations known as "goose flesh" or *cutis anserine*.

Hairs are composed of a cuticle on the outside, usually a medulla in the center and a cortex between the two. Hair is intermittently shed and replaced, hair on the head having a life span of two to four years, while eyelashes have only three to five months.

SEBACEOUS GLANDS

The sebaceous glands are largest and most numerous in the scalp, forehead, cheeks and chin. None are found on the palms and soles, nor on the dorsum of the foot. These glands are large and numerous on the midline of the back, are largest on the face and around the genitalia. Some sebaceous glands open directly onto the surface of the skin, and are found in the palpebrae (Meibomian glands) in the buccal mucosa and the vermilion surface of the lips, on the nipples, on the prepuce (Tyson's glands), occasionally on the glans penis and on the labia minora.

Most sebaceous glands are appendages of hair follicles and open inside the pilosebaceous canal, the size varying inversely with the size of the hair follicles with which they are associated, the largest found on the ala of the nose where hair follicles are small or absent, the hairs being accessories to the glands. In the newborn the glands are large, but they become small shortly after birth, remain small through infancy and childhood, and develop fully in prepuberal years. Larger in men than in women, the glands vary from 0.2 to 2 mm in diameter.

ECCRINE SWEAT GLANDS

Over the general body eccrine sweat glands are most numerous in man, having over two million glands, with an average distribution of about 2800 to the square inch.

Eccrine glands first appear in the fourth fetal month in the palms and soles, appearing in the axilla in the fifth fetal month.

From the latter part of the fifth fetal month they appear over the parts of the skin, arranged in characteristic patterns around hair follicles. These glands are simple tubes that extend from the epidermis to midway in the dermis, or to the tela subcutanea; thus, they are separable into two groups, shallow glands and deep-lying glands.

Eccrine glands are active or inactive. External factors alone are not sufficient to cause sweating. Heat, emotional stresses and sensory stimulation cause sweating, as do gustatory stimulation and muscular exercises, resulting from a combination of thermal and psychic stimulation.

APOCRINE GLANDS

In man, apocrine sweat glands occur in the axilla, the mons pubis, the external auditory meatus, the eyelids, the circumanal area, the areola and nipple of the breast and the labia minora of the female, and in the prepuce and scrotum of the male. "Ectopic" glands may also be found in the face, the scalp and on the abdomen and around the umbilicus.

Apocrine glands grow from the side of hair follicles as solid epithelial buds above the sebaceous glands after the development of the eccrine gland in the fetus after the fifth fetal month.

Secretory process: The orifices of most apocrine glands open inside the pilosebaceous canals or to the surface near the pilosebaceous orifice. Occasionally, the apocrine glands open directly onto the surface of the epidermis.

SURGICAL PROCEDURES
INTEGUMENTARY SYSTEM

Skin and Subcutaneous Areolar Tissue
Incision
   Drainage of infected steatomas.
   Drainage of furuncle.
   Drainage of carbuncle.
   Drainage of subcutaneous abscess.
   Drainage of pilonidal cyst.
   Drainage of onychia or paraonychia
      and may include partial evulsion of
      a nail.
   Incision and removal of a foreign body
      from the subcutaneous tissue.
   Drainage of hematoma.

Puncture aspiration of abscess or hematoma.

Excision

Biopsy of skin or subcutaneous tissue.

Local destruction of, excision of small neoplastic, cicatricial, inflammatory or congenital lesion of skin or subcutaneous tissue.

Wide excision of lesion of skin or subcutaneous tissue, may include graft or plastic closure.

Lipectomy, an excision of fatty tissue.

Excision of nail, nail bed or nail fold.

Excision of pilonidal cyst or sinus.

Excision of hydradenitis suppurativa.

Excision of post-phlebitic varicose ulcer with graft.

Resection of malignant lesion.

Repair (Plastic Surgery)

Applied in situations where delicate handling of tissues, meticulous closure of wounds in layers, and other time consuming techniques commonly employed by the plastic and reconstructive surgeon are necessarily used to obtain maximum functional and cosmetic results. These include the creation or preparation of the defect and its repair. Also, the excision and /or repair by Z-plasty, rotation flap, advanced flap, double pedicle flap, or other rearrangement and suturing of adjacent tissues. Grafting consists of skin grafts, pinch or split skin, 2 to 32 square inches; some procedures requiring skin graft of local flaps to repair donor site; direct flap or tube pedicle formation; delay, intermediate transfer, or sectioning of pedicle or tube graft.

Also, remission, defatting or rearrangement of transferred skin graft procedures are necessary.

Composite Graft: A plastic repair or reconstruction of the full thickness of the external ear or nasal ala.

Debridement, extensive abrasion of wounds.

Abrasion of skin, face for removal of scars, traumatic, tattoos, etc.

Derma, fat, fascia, graft.

Dermabrasion.

Facial injuries and fractures.

Burns

Dressings

Initial or subsequent, large or with major debridement.

Destruction

Cauterization or fulguration of local lesion.

Breast

Incision

Puncture aspiration of cyst.

Mastotomy: Surgical incision of a mamma (mammary gland).

Abscess.

Excision

Breast biopsy.

Excision of cyst, fibroadenoma or other benign tumor, aberrant breast tissue, duct lesion or nipple, and including a partial mastectomy, lateral or bilateral.

Excision of chest wall tumor involving ribs.

Excision of chest wall tumor involving ribs plus plastic reconstruction.

Mastectomy: Excision of a breast.

Radical Mastectomy: Excision of a breast including pectoral muscles and axillary lymph nodes.

Repair

Mastoplasty: A plastic operation on breast, lateral or bilateral.

MUSCULAR SYSTEM

. . . All the body fitly framed and knit together, through that which every joint supplieth . . . EPHESIANS 4, 16

FASCIA

The fibrous connective tissue sheet which covers the body beneath the skin, other than tendons, aponeuroses and ligaments, and which encloses muscles and certain organs is known as *fascia*. Fascia is of three types: *Superficial fascia, deep fascia* and *subserous fascia. Superficial fascia (tela subcutanea)* is continuous over the entire body between the skin and the deep fascial enclosure of the specialized structures of the body, e.g., the muscles. *Deep fascia* immediately covers the muscles composed of intricate series of sheets and bands which holds the muscles and other structures in their proper relative positions. *Subserous* or *visceral fascia* lies between the internal enveloping layer of *deep fascia* and the serous membranes lining the body cavities. This fascia is thin in some areas such as between the pleura and the chest wall, and thick in other areas.

MUSCLES

Muscle tissue provides man with the power of movement. Motion, the important activity of the body is made possible by special development of the function of contractility in muscle tissue. Motion in this sense includes not only movements of the entire body from place to place, but those of breathing, the beating of the heart, movements of the parts of the alimentary tract and its glands, and movements of the other viscera, including those of the blood and lymph vessels.

In man, striated, voluntary or skeletal muscle constitutes 20 to 30 per cent of the body weight.

Special characteristics of muscle tissue are irritability (excitability), contractility, extensibility and elasticity. Irritability, or excitability, is the function of receiving stimuli and responding to them. Contractility is the means which enables muscles to change their shape and become shorter and thicker. Extensibility of a living muscle cell means that it can be stretched or extended; and elasticity means that it readily returns to its original form when the stretching force is removed.

Muscle tissue is composed of long cylindrical fibers or muscle cells, containing several nuclei and embedded in a thin ground substance. These fibers are marked by transverse lines, striated or striped muscle; involuntary muscle consists of long, spindle-shaped uninuclear cells held together by a delicate connective tissue membrane. Connective tissue is the supporting

or framework tissue of the body formed of cells and intercellular substance.

Muscular tissue is classified according to its type or location:

Type	*Location*
Striated, or voluntary	Skeletal
Unstriated, or involuntary	Visceral
Cardiac	Heart

Striated, voluntary or skeletal muscular tissue is termed striated because of the microscopic parallel stripes, or striae; skeletal because it forms the muscles which are attached to the skeleton; and voluntary because the movements accomplished are usually under conscious control.

Unstriated or involuntary muscle which is so-called because it does not exhibit microscopic cross stripes or striae, and is found in the walls of viscera, vessels and glands, in the iris and ciliary muscle, etc., are not under the control of the will, but rather sustain a slow response to the autonomic nervous system.

Cardiac muscle has indistinctly striated muscle tissue which forms the heart. Transverse striations are less distinct than in the skeletal muscles and the cells are smaller. Physiologically one might say the heart action is myogenic in that it has an automatic, rhythmic contraction which, while modified by it, is not initiated by nervous impulses.

Skeletal muscles are arranged in groups with specific functions to perform: (1) flexion and extension, or bending and straightening of a part; (2) external and internal rotation; and (3) abduction away from, and adduction toward, the central axis of the body.

Muscles are named from their shape, size, structure, situation, direction, action and attachment. Many skeletal muscles bear two names, one Latin, and the other English, e.g., obliquus externus abdominis and external abdominal oblique. Sometimes a muscle has more than one Latin name, e.g., psoas magnus and psoas major, vastus intermedius and vastus crureus. Frequently a muscle has no well known English name, e.g., levatores costarum; sometimes the English name is the one that is best known, e.g., deltoid instead of deltoideus, e.g., pterygoideus externus and pterygoideus internus and pterygoideus medialis.

Each muscle has motor and sensory nerve fibers and is well supplied with arteries, capillaries, veins and lymphatics. The points of attachment of a muscle are its origin and insertion. The attachment to the more movable part of the skeleton is the insertion; thus, when a muscle contracts, insertion moves towards the origin. The more fixed attachment serves as the basis of action and is the origin of the muscle. There are over 600 named muscles of the body (Plates 11-17) and some of these are classified below:

MUSCLES OF EXPRESSION

Epicranial	Platysma
Corrugator	Risorius
Buccinator	Quadrati labii
Zygomatic	Mentalis
Triangularis	Nasal muscles
	Orbicularis oris

This group of muscles enables one to express pleasure, pain, disgust, disdain, contempt, fear, anger, sadness, surprise, or other emotional states.

MUSCLE MOVEMENT

MOVEMENT OF EYE AND LIDS

Movement of the eyeball is controlled by six muscles. The orbit contains seven muscles; six of them are attached to the eyeball, arranged in three opposing pairs, levator, palpebrae, superioris, orbicularis oculi and corrugator.

MUSCLES OF MASTICATION

The muscles of mastication are the masseter (chewing muscle), the temporal (temple muscle), the internal pterygoid and the external pterygoid.

MOVEMENT OF HEAD

Flexion	Extension
Sternocleidomastoid	Splenius capitis
	Semispinalis capitis
	Longissimus capitis

MOVEMENT OF VERTEBRAL COLUMN

Flexion	Extension
Quadratus lumborum	Sacrospinalis

Forward and backward movement of the spine is limited in the thoracic region but movement is free in the lumbar region, particularly between the fourth and fifth lumbar vertebrae.

MOVEMENT OF SHOULDER GIRDLE

Elevation	Depression
Levator scapulae	Pectoralis minor
Rhomboideus major	Subclavius
Rhomboideus minor	Trapezius (lower fibers)
Trapezius (upper fibers)	

MOVEMENT OF HUMERUS

Flexion	Extension
Coracobrachialis	Teres major

Abduction	Adduction
Deltoid	Pectoralis major
Supraspinatus	

External Rotation	Internal Rotation
Infraspinatus	Latissimus dorsi
Teres Minor	

MOVEMENT BETWEEN HUMERUS AND ULNA

Flexion	Extension
Brachiolis	Triceps
Biceps brachii	
Brachioradialis	

MOVEMENT AT RADIOULNAR JOINT
Movement of Hand

Supination	Pronation
Biceps brachii	Pronator teres
Supinator (brevis)	Pronator quadratus

Movement of Wrist

Flexion	Extension
Flexor carpi radialis	Extensor carpi radialis longus
Flexor carpi ulnaris	Extensor carpi ulnaris

Movement of Fingers

Flexion	Extension
Flexor digitorum profundus	Extensor digitorum communis
Flexor digitorum sublimis	

Movement of Thumb

Flexion	Extension
Flexor pollicis longus	Extensor pollicis longus

Abduction	Adduction
Abductor pollicis longus	Adductor pollicis obliquus
	Adductor pollicis transver salis

MUSCLES OF RESPIRATION

Inspiration	*Expiration*
Diaphragm	Internal intercostals
External intercostals	Abdominal muscles

MOVEMENT OF FEMUR

Flexion	*Extension*
Psoas major	Gluteus maximus
Iliacus	

Abduction	*Adduction*
Gluteus medius	Adductor magnus
Tensor fasciae latae	Adductor longus
	Adductor brevis

Outward Rotation	*Inward rotation*
Priformis	Gluteus minimus (anterior part)
Quadratus femoris	
Obturators	Gluteus medius (anterior part)

MOVEMENT OF KNEE JOINT

Flexion	*Extension*
Biceps femoris	Quadriceps femoris
Semitendinosus	Rectus femoris
Popliteus	Vastus lateralis
Gracilis	Vastus medialis
Sartorius	Vastus intermedius

MOVEMENT OF FOOT

Plantar Flexion	*Dorsiflexion*
Gastrocnemius	Tibialis anterior
Soleus	Perioneus tertius
Tibialis posterior	

MOVEMENT OF TOES

Flexion	*Extension*
Flexor hallucis longus	Extensor hallucis longus
Flexor digitorum longus	Extensor digitorum

MUSCLES OF SCALP

The skin of the scalp is thicker than on any other part of the body. It is adherent to the superficial fascia, which attaches it firmly to the underlying aponeurosis and muscle. Movements of the muscle move the skin. The hair follicles are closely set together and extend throughout the whole thickness of the skin. It also contains a number of sebaceous glands.

Superficial fascia (tela subcutanea) and muscles of the scalp
> Epicranius, occipitofrontalis, and temporoparietalis (covers the top of the skull)
>
> Occipitalis

Frontalis, connected by an intervening tendinous aponeurosis
Galea aponeurotica
Transversus nuchae—thin muscular slip

MUSCLES OF THE EYELIDS

Levator palpebrae superioris
Orbicularis oculi
Corrugator

MUSCLES OF NOSE

Procerus	Depressor Septi
Nasalis	Dilator Naris Posterior
	Dilator Naris Anterior

MUSCLES OF MOUTH

Quadratus labii superioris	Quadratus labii inferioris
Canionus	Triangularis
Zygomaticus	Buccinator
Mentalis	Orbicularis oris
Masseter	Pterygoideus externus
Temporalis	Pterygoideus internus

ANTEROLATERAL MUSCLES OF NECK

Superficial Cervical (Platysma)	Infrahyoid—Sternohyoideus
Lateral Cervical	Sternothyreohyoideus
Trapezius	Thyreohyoideus
Sternocleidomastoideus	Omohyoideus

Suprahyoid

Digastricus	Mylohyoideus
Stylohyoideus	Geniohyoideus

Anterior Vertebral

Longus Colli	Rectus Capitis Anterior
Longus Capitis	Rectus Capitis Lateralis

Lateral Vertebral

Scalenus anterior	Scalenus medius
	Scalenus posterior

DEEP MUSCLES OF BACK

Splenius Capitis	Multifidus
Splenius Cervicis	Rotatores
Sacrospinalis	Interspinalis
Semispinalis	Intertransversarii

MUSCLES OF THORAX

Intercostales externi	Levatores costarum
Intercostales interni	Serratus posterior superior
Subcostales	Serratus posterior inferior
Transversus thoracis	Diaphragm

MUSCLES OF ABDOMEN

Obliquus externus	Transversus
Obliquus internis	Rectus
Pyramidalis	

MUSCLES OF ABDOMEN
(POSTERIOR)

Psoas major	Iliacus
Psoas minor	Quadratus lumborum

MUSCLES OF PELVIS

Obturator internus	Levator ani
Piriformis	Coccygeus

MUSCLES OF ANAL REGION

Corrugator cutis ani	Sphincter ani externus
	Sphincter ani internus

UROGENITAL REGION IN MALE

Transversus perinaei superficialis	Ischiocavernosus
Bulbocavernosus	Transversus perinaei profundus
	Sphincter urethra membranaceae

MUSCLES OF UPPER EXTREMITY CONNECTING TO VERTEBRAL COLUMN

Trapezius	Rhomboideus major
Latissimus dorsi	Rhomboideus minor
	Levator scapulae

MUSCLES OF ANTERIOR AND LATERAL THORACIC REGION

Pectoralis major	Subclavius
Pectoralis Minor	Serratus anterior

MUSCLES OF SHOULDER

Deltoideus	Infraspinatus
Subscapularis	Teres minor
Supraspinatus	Teres major

MUSCLES OF ARM

Corachobrachialis	Brachialis
Biceps brachii	Triceps Brachii

SUPERFICIAL GROUP

Pronator Teres	Palmaris longus
Flexor carpi radialis	Flexor carpi ulnaris

This group originates from the epicondyle of the humerus by a common tendon receiving additional fibers from the deep fascia of the forearm near the elbow.

DEEP GROUP

Flexor digitorum profundus	Flexor pollicis Longus
	Pronator quadratus

MUSCLES OF HAND

Thenar eminence—thumb (radial side)
Hypothenar—little finger (venar side)

Thenar Muscles

Abductor pollicis brevis	Flexor pollicis brevis
Apponeus pollicis	Adductor pollicis (obliquus)
	Adductor pollicis (transversus)

Hypothenar Muscles

Palmaris brevis	Flexor digiti quinti brevis
Abductor digiti quinti	Apponeus digiti quinti

Intermediate Muscles

Lumbricales	Interossei

MUSCLES OF LOWER EXTREMITY

Iliac Region

Muscles of the psoas major and iliacus are sometimes referred to as the iliopsoas.

Psoas major	Iliacus	Psoas Minor

Thigh—Anterior femoral muscles

Sartorius	Quadriceps] femoris]	Rectus femoris Vastus lateralis
femoris	] Vastus medialis	] Vastus intermedius

Medial Femoral Muscle

Gracilus	Adductor longus
Pectineus	Adductor brevis
	Adductor magnus

MUSCLES OF GLUTEAL REGION

Gluteus maximus	Obturator internus
Gluteus medius	Gemellus superior
Gluteus minimus	Gemellus inferior
Tensor fasciae Latae	Quadratus femoris
Piriformis	Obturator externus

MUSCLES OF LEG

Anterior	Anterior Crural muscles
Posterior	Posterior Crural muscles—
Lateral	superficial and deep

Superficial Group

Gastrocnemius	Plantaris
	Soleus

Deep Group

Popliteus	Flexor digitorum longus
Flexor Hallucis longus	Tibialis posterior
Lateral Crural Muscles	
Peronaeus longus	Peronaeus brevis

Fascia around the ankle comprises three ligaments, i.e., the transverse crural, cruciate crural and the lacinate, together with the superior and inferior peroneal retinacula.

MUSCLES OF FOOT

The muscles are divided into three groups and are similar to those in the hand.
1. Dorsal
2. Plantar
a. First layer
   Abductor hallucis
   Flexor digitorum brevis
   Abductor digiti quinti
b. Second layer
   Quadratus plantae
   Lumbricales
c. Third layer
   Flexor hallicus brevis
   Adductor hallucis
   Flexor digiti quinti brevis
d. Fourth layer
   Interossei dorsales (dorsal interossei)
   Interossei plantares (plantar interossei)

SURGICAL PROCEDURES— MUSCLES

Fascia

Incision
   Fasciotomy: surgical incision of a fascia.
   Removal of foreign body in muscle with general anesthesia.
   Division of scalenus anticus, with or without resection of cervical rib.
   Division of sternomastoid for torticollis open operation.
Suture
   Fasciorrhaphy: suturing together of torn fascia.

Tendons, Tendon Sheaths and Fascia

Incision
   Drainage of tendon sheath, infection for acute tenosynovitis, by digits.
   Drainage of tendon sheath, infection for acute tenosynovitis, single palm or wrist, ulnar or radical bursa infection.
   Injection of medication into tendon sheath or hand.
   Incision of fibrous sheath of tendon for stenosing tenosynovitis, to include freeing of tendons or removal of foreign body.
   Division of iliotibial band, open operation.

Stripping of ilium (Souter operation)
Tenotomy: division of a tendon, particularly for strabismius or club foot.
Fasciotomy: for Dupuytren's contracture, partial including finger extensions and vertical bands, radical.
Excision
   Tendonectomy: excision of portion of a tendon to shorten it.
   Excision of small ganglion cyst.
   Tenosynovectomy: excision or resection of tendon sheath.
   Excision of lesion of tendon or fibrous sheath, including ganglion, digits only or in other locations.
   Radical excision of bursae, forearm, viz. tenosynovitis fungosa, Tbs., and other granulomas.
   Excision of Barker's cyst (synovial cyst of popliteal space).
Repair
   Fascioplasty: any plastic operation on the fascia.
   Repair or suture extensor tendon, single, hand or foot, distal to wrist or ankle single, forearm or leg.
   Repair or suture flexor tendon, single.
   Transfer, or transplant, or free graft of tendon, single, distal to elbow, or distal to knee; single, elbow to shoulder, or knee to hip.
   Tenomyoplasty: plastic operation involving tendon and muscle.
   Tenolysis: lengthening or shortening of a tendon.
   Retrieve or rerouting of a tendon through a separate incision.
   Free fascial graft for reconstruction of a tendon pulley, or repairing a bowstring tendon.
   Repair bowstring tendon to form gliding surface for tendons.
   Abdominal fascial transplants, bilateral.
   Free fascial graft to face.
   Patellar advancement.
   Rupture quadriceps insertion.
   Rupture biceps tendon from insertion, elbow.
   Flexor plasty elbow.
   Repair ruptured supraspinatus tendon or musculotendinous shoulder cuff.
Suture.

Suture of complete shoulder cuff avulsion.

Tenorrhaphy: surgical union of a divided tendon.

Extremities

Incision

Drainage of felon in hospital with general anesthetic.

Drainage of single, infected space of hand (lumbrical, hypothenar, thenar, middle palmar, etc.) with or without tendon sheath involvement.

Drainage of multiple infected spaces of hand (with or without tendon sheath involvement).

NERVOUS SYSTEM

My skull teems with notions infinite. CHARLES LAMB

Activities of even the smallest communities must be coordinated by a central authority towards a common goal. God solved this problem within man by creating a controlling system, the nervous system (our electrical wiring system).

In its simplest form the nervous system is merely a mechanism by which a muscular movement can be initiated by some change in peripheral sensation, such as an object touching the skin. It is concerned with the correlation and integration of bodily processes, the sensations and adjustments to its environment and with conscious life.

The nervous system is divided into three categories. However, it is emphasized that all of these divisions are merely arbitrary and artificial, remembering their essential unity in structure and their interdependence in function. These three categories are:
1. Central nervous system
   (1) Brain, encephalon
   (2) Spinal Cord, medulla spinalis
2. Peripheral nervous system
   (1) Cerebrospinal nerves
      (a) Cranial nerves
      (b) Spinal nerves
3. Autonomic nervous system
   (1) Sympathetic nervous system
   (2) Parasympathetic nervous system
      (a) Preganglian
      (b) Postganglian

These complicated systems are composed of large numbers of essentially integral units called neurons, the fundamental unit of nervous tissue composed of a cell body together with its process, dendrites and axons especially adapted to carry a message or impulse rapidly over considerable distances, in some instances up to four feet in length. Neurons conduct impulses in a chain-type sequence, traveling in only one direction made possible by the minute gap between the neurons, called synapses. Nerve stations or synapses transmit the nervous impulse from the first to the second neuron forming short or long nerve pathways.

Somatic (concerned with reactions to the changing conditions of the environment) afferent (incoming) nerve fibers transmit sensation from the body to the spinal cord, comprising those sensations of exteroception, such as pain, temperature, touch and pressure. Proprioceptive sensations also included are sensations from muscles, tendons and joints providing information on joint position, and the tension of tendons and muscle fibers.

Visceral (concerned with maintenance within the body of conditions suitable to life) afferent nerve fibers convey impulses from mucous membranes, glands and blood vessels.

Somatic efferent (outgoing) nerve fibers carry motor impulses to skeletal muscles.

Visceral efferent nerve fibers supply smooth muscle and glandular tissues.

Specific function and direction of conduction provided by these terminal features of the nerve fiber and the pattern organization of the synapses which a nerve impulse may follow in the central nervous system, gives the brain and spinal cord its particular contribution to the body as a whole.

Each neuron has a distinct polarity. The unipolar cells are those having a single process, and are found in the spinal ganglia. Bipolar cells are those having processes extending from either end of the cell, and are found in the sympathetic ganglia. (The ganglionated sympathetic trunks lie parallel to the vertebral column and are connected with each pair of the 31 spinal nerves and with nerves and ganglia of the viscera.) The multipolar cells are pyramidal in shape, with many processes leaving at various places, and are found in the brain and spinal cord. Another main element of nervous tissue is the neuroglia, which is similar to connective tissue in function, thus supporting the nerve cells.

Nerve fiber is composed of axons and their associated structures. The axon or core of the nerve fiber, also known as the axis cylinder or neuraxon, is covered by a fatty myelin sheath, and this is in turn surrounded by a nucleated layer of tissue, the neurilemma. At regular intervals there are interruptions, the nodes of Ranvier, which divide the fiber into segments. This fiber is known as medullated or myelinated fiber and is white. Another type of fiber is known as unmyelinated or nonmedullated fiber, gray or yellow in color, and does not have a myelin sheath.

Neurons carrying impulses to the center are known as receptor, sensory or afferent. Neurons carrying impulses from the center to the periphery are known as effector, motor or efferent. Neurons carrying impulses from afferent to efferent neurons are known as internuncial, connecting or central associations. Nerves are composed of either sensory or motor fibers; if these contain both, they are referred to as mixed fibers.

Bundles of nerve fibers are gathered together by a connective tissue sheath, the endoneurium, which forms the fasciculi or funiculi, the nerve tracts. These are held together by connective tissue, the perineurium, and surrounded by a sheath called the epineurium. The fasciculi form a nerve trunk; thus, nerves are branches of nerve trunks. The nerve trunk at intervals has visible bulges composed of masses of cell bodies which are named according to their location. The ganglion is the name of the mass lying outside the brain and spinal cord; nucleus is the mass found inside the substance of the brain or spinal cord.

While cranial nerves exhibit the funda-mental components, the types of sensation are designated as "special." Such special somatic afferent nerve fibers involve those nerves serving the special senses of vision and hearing; special senses of visceral afferent nerve fibers transmit impulses of taste and smell.

Nerve fibers are therefore the conducting elements of the nerve cell or neuron, sending an impulse in any direction. The motor endplate termination of a motor nerve gives it its specific function. Specificity then is determined in the nerve fibers by its termination, i.e., a "pain" fiber conducts painful impulses because of its freely branched ending in the epidermis of the skin. Each nerve is a collection of nerve fibers which conduct various types of sensation, and impulses passing to muscles or gland cells.

CENTRAL NERVOUS SYSTEM

BRAIN

The brain is defined anatomically as that part of the nervous system which lies within the cranial cavity of the skull. It is a suprasegmented monitoring apparatus concerned with all somatic and visceral functions. It serves as a center for integrating responses to sensory stimuli arriving by way of the ascending tracts of the spinal cord and cranial nerves. It arises in the embryo as a development of the head end of the neural tube.

The brain lies within and nearly fills the cranial cavity. It is continuous through the foramen magnum with the spinal cord, which occupies but does not fill the spinal canal. From the brain arises a series of nerves usually enumerated as 12 pairs and known as cranial or cerebral nerves.

Parts of the brain are medulla, pons, midbrain, interbrain (or diencephalon), cerebellum, cerebrum and meninges. The *medulla* lies between the spinal cord and the pons. The *pons* consists of a bridge of fibers that connect the halves of the cerebellum and join the midbrain above with the medulla below. The *midbrain* is composed of the corpora quadrigemina and the cerebral peduncles. The former (quadrigemina) serve as relay centers for the visual and auditory reflexes; the latter are composed of bundles of fibers that form conducting pathways for impulses to and from the cerebrum. The *cerebellum* serves as a reflex center through which muscular movements maintaining posture and equilibrium are coordinated. The *cerebrum* is divided into right and left hemispheres by the great longitudinal fissure. Each hemisphere is divided into five lobes; frontal, parietal, temporal, occipital, and insula.

Functions localized in definite regions of the cerebral cortex are motor, sensory, auditory, visual, speech and olfactory areas. It is assumed that the remaining portions are concerned with intellectual processes involving memory, reason and judgment.

The thalamus is a relay station for impulses passing to and from the cerebral cortex, and serves as a center of primitive sensation. The hypothalamus contains the temperature-regulating centers; through connections with the pituitary gland, it plays an important part in the regulation of water, fat and carbohydrate metabolism. It is a coordinating center for the autonomic nervous system.

The reticular formation forms the central core of the brain stem. One of the more important integrating structures in the central nervous system, it influences perception, arousal, wakefulness and motor functions in muscular control.

The three membranes investing the brain and spinal cord are the dura mater (external), the arachnoid (middle) and the pia mater (internal).

Dura mater is adherent to the inner surface of the cranium where it serves the double function of an internal periosteum and a covering for the brain. Two conspicuous folds of the dura mater, the falx cerebri and the tentorium cerebelli, are given off from the deep surface. The *falx cerebri* is a sickle-shaped partition which passes in the greater longitudinal fissure between the hemispheres. Its inferior border arches over the corpus callosum. The *tentorium cerebelli* forms a roof for the posterior cranial cavity and separates the cerebellum from the posterior part of the cerebrum. The dura mater, or outermost of these covering layers, is divided into two layers which separate along certain lines to form venous channels or sinuses for the passage of blood

from the brain. The more important sinuses are the superior sagittal sinus along the superior border of the falx cerebri, the inferior sagittal sinus on the inferior border, the straight sinus where the falx cerebri joins the tentorium, the transverse sinus along the occipital and temporal bones, and the cavernous sinus in the region of the sella turcica.

The *arachnoid* is a fine membrane loosely disposed over the surface of the brain. It does not dip down into the sulci between convolutions. The arachnoid membrane forms finger-like projections, called villi, which penetrate the walls of the sinuses and extend into them. The subarachnoid space, like its counterpart in the spinal cord, contains cerebrospinal fluid.

Pia mater, or the innermost of these covering layers, is closely adherent to the surface of the brain and is carried down into the sulci between convolutions. The ependyma lines the ventricules and forms the choroid plexuses of these spaces. Close association of some arachnoid and pia mater may be referred to as the leptomeninges.

SPINAL CORD

The spinal cord, or medulla spinalis, is a cylindrical mass of nervous tissue occupying the upper two-thirds of the spinal canal. It is composed of 31 segments of nervous tissue, each bearing a pair of spinal nerves. The spinal cord is 18 inches (40 to 50 cm) in length. It is continuous with the medulla oblongata of the brain stem at the foramen magnum, and inferiorly extends to the level of the upper border of the second lumbar vertebra. The lower end tapers off to a point and is called the *conus medullaris* and is continued in a mixed nervous and pia strand, the filum terminale. The filum terminale descends, becomes invested by the coccygeal ligament of dura mater, and together with it attaches to the tip of the coccyx.

Even above this level the vertebral canal is by no means fully occupied by the spinal cord, being surrounded by the pia mater, the cerebrospinal fluid, the arachnoid and the dura mater, which later fuses with the periosteum of the inner surfaces of the vertebrae.

The disparity between the length of the spinal cord and spinal canal increases the distance between the attachment of the various nerve roots and the intervertebral foramina through which the several nerves leave the vertebral canal. Therefore, the nerve roots arising from the lumbar and sacral region pass for some distance in the canal before making their exit. This bundle of nerve roots is called the *cauda equina.*

Immediately surrounding the brain and cord and adherent to them is the delicate, highly vascular pia mater. This is separated from the thick, fibroid dura mater by a membrane having the tenuity of a spider web, the arachnoid, which surrounds the subarachnoid space. This space is broken up by subarachnoid trabeculae and filled with cerebrospinal fluid. Between the arachnoid, which, although thin, is a complete membrane, and the dura mater lies the subdural space, which normally contains only enough fluid to moisten the surfaces. There is no communication between the subarachnoid and subdural spaces. In spinal punctures, the needle must traverse the subdural space to enter the subarachnoid space where the cerebrospinal fluid is found. Cerebrospinal fluid is a clear, slightly viscous liquid circulating in the subarachnoid space about the brain and spinal cord.

The spinal cord serves as a center for spinal reflexes and as a pathway for nerve impulses passing to and from the brain. The cord consists of a central core of gray matter surrounded by white matter.

The spinal cord and attached nerve roots within the vertebral canal are also surrounded by three coverings: dura mater, arachnoid and pia mater.

Reflexes may involve only one level of the spinal cord, or the impulses may spread upward or downward through internuncial neurons, producing an almost infinite variety of responses.

Reflexes that can be elicited in the isolated spinal cord include the stretch reflex, the flexion reflex, crossed-extension reflex and certain long spinal reflexes.

Transections of the spinal cord result in immediate and permanent loss of all sensation and all capability of voluntary movement below the level of the transection.

The spinal cord contains a butterfly-shaped area of gray matter surrounded by an area of white matter. The white matter consists primarily of ascending and descending nerve fibers, serving as our conducting pathway for long or short impulses. Some of these may ascend or descend a short distance to accomplish a broader reflex within a few segments of the spinal cord; however, others ascend to carry sensory impulses to higher centers of the brain, or descend from the brain to initiate willed action, indicating, therefore, that the spinal cord reflex is influenced by other brain mechanisms at all times.

PERIPHERAL NERVOUS SYSTEM
CEREBROSPINAL NERVES

The cerebrospinal nerves form a part of the peripheral portion of the nervous system. Cerebrospinal nerves, as the name implies, include the cranial and spinal nerves.

Cranial Nerves

The cranial nerves are designated as those, attached to the brain, which pass through the foramina of the skull. Twelve pairs symmetrically arranged are distributed mainly to the structure of the head and neck (Plates 18 and 19). Because of the diversity of their function, the nerves have been given names as well as numbers. The sensory components have their cell bodies in ganglia outside the brain; the cell bodies of the motor components are in the nuclei of the brain.

I. Olfactory Nerves (Sensory) or Nerves of Smell: The olfactory nerve fibers are the central processes (axons) of the spindle-shaped, bipolar cell bodies situated in the olfactory region of the nasal cavity of the nose.

II. Optic (Sensory): The optic nerve is the special nerve of the sense of sight. It consists of fibers derived from ganglionic cells of the retina.

III. Oculomotor nerve (Motor): This nerve contains somatic motor fibers for innervation of the Levator palpebra and all but two of the extrinsic muscles of the eye except the obliquus superioris and rectus lateralis. The *oculomotor nerve* also contains autonomic fibers for the ciliaris muscle, sphincter pupillae and proprioceptive fibers from the above extrinsic muscles.

IV. Trochear Nerve (Motor): This is the smallest of the cranial nerves. It supplies muscle sense and the impulse for movement to the superior oblique muscle of the eye.

V. Trigeminal Nerve (Mixed) or Trifacial Nerve: This is the largest of the cranial nerves. It is composed of a large sensory root and a smaller motor root. It is sometimes referred to as the great sensory nerve of the head and face because it supplies the sense of touch, pain, heat and cold to the skin of the face and scalp and the mucous membranes of the head.

VI. Abducens Nerve (Motor): This cranial nerve completes the innervation of the extrinsic eye muscles by supplying afferent and efferent fibers to the lateral rectus muscle for muscle sense and motion.

VII. Facial Nerve (Mixed): The facial or seventh nerve consists of motor and sensory divisions; of the two, the motor (in contrast to the fifth) is the larger, supplying motor fibers to the muscles of the face, scalp and auricle. The sensory part contains the fibers of taste for the anterior two-thirds of the tongue.

VIII. Acoustic Nerve (Sensory): This cranial nerve has two distinct parts known as the vestibular and cochlear nerves. Both divisions are confined to carrying impulses for sensation from the inner ear. The vestibular nerve mediates the impulses for equilibriation. The cochlear nerve is known as the nerve of hearing.

IX. Glossopharyngeal Nerve (Mixed): The glossopharyngeal nerve provides for reflex control of the tongue, taste and swallowing reflexes. These impulses are initiated by stimulation of the carotid sinus, taste-buds, of the posterior third of the tongue, and mucous membrane of the pharynx, soft palate and tonsils.

X. Vagus Nerve (Mixed): This, the tenth cranial nerve, has the most extensive distribution of any in this series since it passes through the neck and goes to structures in the thorax to the abdomen, as well as in the head and neck.

The afferent impulses are obtained from the mucous membrane of the larynx, trachea and bronchi, lungs, arch of the aorta, esophagus and stomach. Efferent impulses affect gastric secretion, for example.

It is through this innervation that the reflex control of respiratory rate, and accessory respiratory reflexes (coughing and sneezing), reflex inhibition of heart rate and the sensation of hunger are facilitated.

XI. Accessory Nerve (Motor): The eleventh cranial nerve consists of cranial and spinal divisions. Afferent and efferent spinal components carry muscle sense and motor impulses for the sternocleidomastoid and trapezius muscles. Entering the skull through the jugular foramen, afferent fibers terminate and efferent fibers arise in the medulla and cervical spinal cord. The medullary components leave the accessory nerve to become a portion of the vagus nerve as both nerves emerge from the jugular foramen.

XII. Hypoglossal Nerve (Motor): From the medulla, the hypoglossal nerve runs dorsal to the vertebral artery through the hypo-glossal foramen to the inferior surface of the tongue. Both muscle sense and motion are provided for the muscles of the tongue by this nerve.

Spinal Nerves

The 31 pairs of spinal nerves correspond to segments of the spinal cord, and are classified as 8 cervical, 12 thoracic, 5 lumbar, 5 sacral and 1 coccygeal. They are formed by the fibers from the dorsal and ventral roots which join as they pass out through the intervertebral foramen. The spinal nerves each continue for only a few millimeters before dividing into anterior and posterior branches. In general, the posterior division supplies the muscles of the back acting on the vertebral column and the skin covering them. The anterior division is large and forms the main portion of the spinal nerve. It supplies the muscles, skin of the extremities and the remaining area of the trunk (Plates 20-22).

AUTONOMIC NERVOUS SYSTEM

By definition, the term "autonomic" implies self-control and independence of outside influences, and as a result has sometimes been given the alternate names of involuntary or vegetative nervous system.

The autonomic nervous system is an aggregation of ganglia, nerves and plexuses through which the viscera, glands, heart and blood vessels, as well as smooth muscle in other situations, receive their innervation. It is widely distributed over the body, especially in the head and neck and in the thoracic and abdominal cavities. It is divided into a craniosacral (parasympathetic) division and a thoracolumbar (sympathetic) division, the portions of the central nervous system to which each is related. Parasympathetic stimulation slows the heart rate, and sympathetic stimulation increases the heart rate.

The autonomic nervous system governs the activities of such visceral structures as heart, lungs, digestive tube, glands, blood vessels, uterus, urinary bladder and certain endocrine glands. This system performs the important function of maintaining the constancy of composition of the internal environment and through its manifold activities works to resist forces that tend to alter the internal environment.

Regulation of the body fluids in respect to composition, temperature quantity and distribution is brought about through the action of this system on circulatory, respiratory, excretory and glandular organs; e.g., the liver, pancreas and adrenals, which are controlled by autonomic influence, are important in regulation of blood sugar, sweat glands and in the control of temperature, and the regulation of heart action and of the caliber of blood vessels, and thereby determine the distribution of the internal environment.

Most visceral structures receive fibers from both divisions of the autonomic system and effects exerted by the two types of fibers on a given organ are antagonistic. Thus the heart rate is slowed by the craniosacral division (vagus) and accelerated by the thoracolumbar division.

The most conspicuous parts of the autonomic system are the sympathetic trunks —two nerve cords extending vertically through the neck, thorax and abdomen, one on each side of the vertebral column. Each trunk is composed of a series of ganglia arranged in linear order and bound together by short nerve strands.

It has been customary to consider visceral innervation under the heading of sympathetic nervous system, as if it were something which acted companionably but apart from the rest of the nervous system.

Thus, the 12 pairs of cranial nerves supply structures of the head and neck region. The vagus nerve passes into the thorax and abdomen to the viscera.

In general, the craniosacral system is concerned with conservative and restorative processes, while the thoracolumbar division governs processes involving an expenditure of energy.

In the craniosacral division the slowing of the heart rate, constriction of coronary arteries, contraction of the pupil, for protection of the eye from intense light, action of the liver, inhibiting glycogen mobilization, and effects on the gastrointestinal tract favoring digestion and absorption through which energy supplies are stored all furnish evidence of the conservative activities controlled by this division.

The thoracolumbar division has been called the emergency mechanism of the body because it is brought into activity by conditions that call for "fright or flight."

Structurally, each portion of the autonomic system consists of two-neuron chains. The first neuron, or preganglionic neuron, has its cell body in the visceral efferent (nerve) column of the brain or spinal cord. The second neuron, or postganglionic neuron, has its cell body in the ganglion outside of the cerebrospinal axis.

In the craniosacral (parasympathetic) division, preganglionic neurons begin in the nuclei of origin of cranial nerves III, VII, IX and X and in the second, third and fourth sacral segments of the spinal cord.

In this division the preganglionic neurons follow the spinal nerves indistinguishably into their peripheral distribution.

In the thoracolumbar (sympathetic) division the preganglionic neurons are located in the spinal cord beginning at the first thoracic level and end at the second and third lumbar level.

The sympathetic portion of the system innervates all smooth muscle and glands of the body, and striated muscle of the heart.

Stratified squamous epithelium; serves as protection; covers the body forming the epithelium and is found wherever the ectoderm folds in, e.g. mouth, nose, and anus.

 Ciliated epithelium; lines the respiratory pathway from the nose to the bronchial tubes (with the exception of the pharynx and vocal cords).

 Striated muscle; moves the body.

 Cardiac muscle; acts as a pump to keep blood moving.

 Areolar connective tissue; has many functions; stores 15% of body water

 Adipose tissue; pads, protects and stores fat.

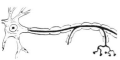 Motor nerve cell; the nervous system is made up of countless numbers of these cells.

 Hyaline cartilage; forms part of skeletal framework.

 Haversian system of compact bone.

 Section of stomach; secretes gastric juice.

 Section of duodenum; secretes digestive fluids, absorbs the nutrients from foods.

 Section of colon.

 Liver - chain of cells; has many important functions essential to life.

 Pancreas; secretes digestive fluids.

Plates 1 and 2. Unit patterns and tissue relationships of the body. (From Kimber, D. C., Stackpole, C. E., Gray, C. E., and Leavell, L. C.: *Textbook of Anatomy and Physiology*, Ed. 14. The Macmillan Company, New York, 1961. Reprinted with the permission of The Macmillan Company.)

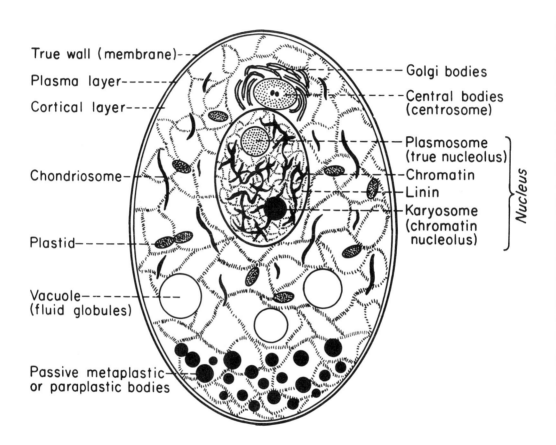

True wall (membrane)

Plasma layer

Cortical layer

Chondriosome

Plastid

Vacuole
(fluid globules)

Passive metaplastic
or paraplastic bodies

Golgi bodies

Central bodies
(centrosome)

Plasmosome
(true nucleolus)

Chromatin

Linin

Karyosome
(chromatin
nucleolus)

Nucleus

Plate 3. Diagram of a cell

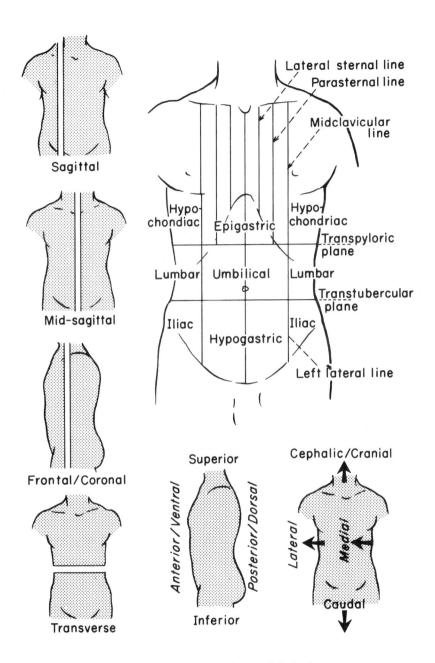

Plate 4. Anatomical positions of the body

The <u>dorsal</u> <u>cavity</u> is divided into:
  The <u>cranial</u> <u>cavity</u> containing the brain,
  and the <u>vertebral</u> <u>cavity</u> containing the
  spinal cord.

The <u>ventral</u> <u>cavity</u> is divided into:
  The <u>thoracic</u> and <u>abdominopelvic</u>
  <u>cavities</u>.

The <u>abdominopelvic</u> <u>cavity</u> is subdivided
  into the <u>abdominal</u> <u>portion</u> containing
  the liver, gallbladder, stomach, spleen,
  pancreas, and small and large intes-
  tines ; and the <u>pelvic</u> <u>portion</u> containing the bladder, rectum, sigmoid colon
  and reproductive organs.

The <u>thoracic</u> <u>cavity</u> is subdivided
  into the right and left <u>pleural</u>
  <u>cavities</u> containing the lungs,
  and the <u>mediastinum</u> which contains
  all other thoracic viscera including
  the heart enclosed in the <u>pericardial</u>
  <u>cavity</u>.

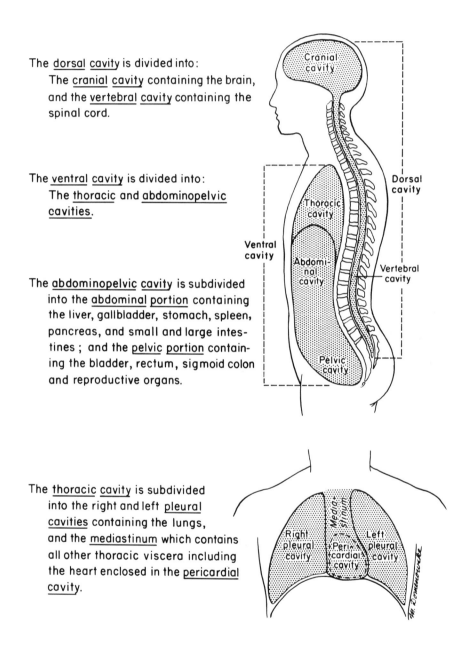

Plate 5. Cavities of the body

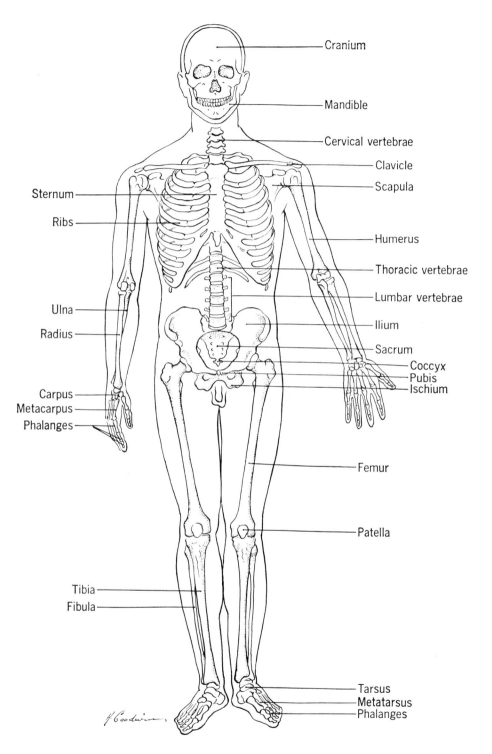

Plate 6. Human skeleton, anterior view. (Reprinted from *Stedman's Medical Dictionary*, Ed. 20. The Williams & Wilkins Co., Baltimore, 1961.)

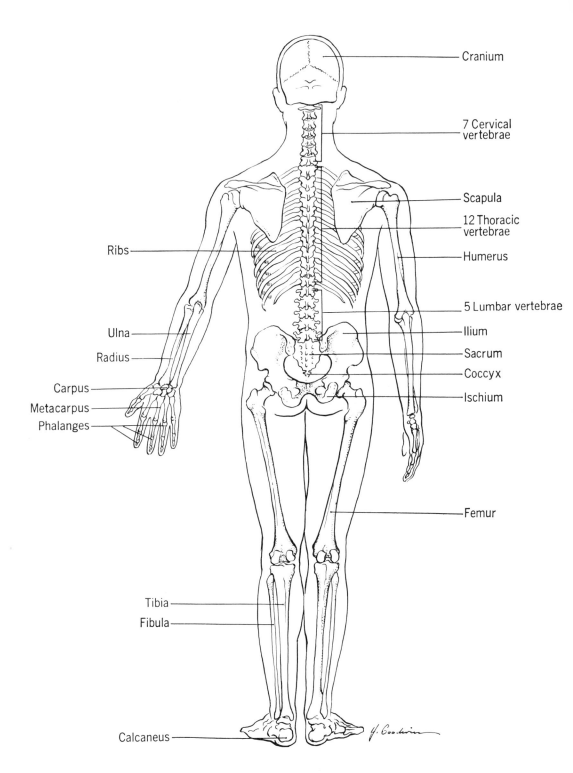

Cranium

7 Cervical vertebrae

Scapula

12 Thoracic vertebrae

Humerus

5 Lumbar vertebrae

Ilium

Sacrum

Coccyx

Ischium

Ribs

Ulna

Radius

Carpus

Metacarpus

Phalanges

Femur

Tibia

Fibula

Calcaneus

Plate 7. Human skeleton, posterior view. (Reprinted from *Stedman's Medical Dictionary*, Ed. 20. The Williams & Wilkins Co., Baltimore, 1961.)

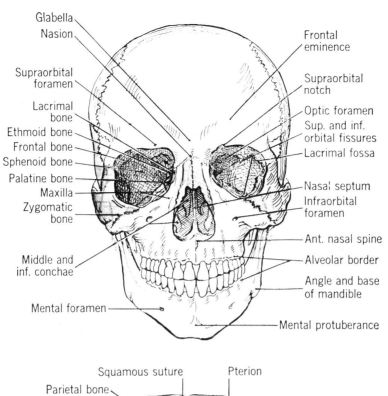

Glabella
Nasion
Supraorbital foramen
Lacrimal bone
Ethmoid bone
Frontal bone
Sphenoid bone
Palatine bone
Maxilla
Zygomatic bone
Middle and inf. conchae
Mental foramen

Frontal eminence
Supraorbital notch
Optic foramen
Sup. and inf. orbital fissures
Lacrimal fossa
Nasal septum
Infraorbital foramen
Ant. nasal spine
Alveolar border
Angle and base of mandible
Mental protuberance

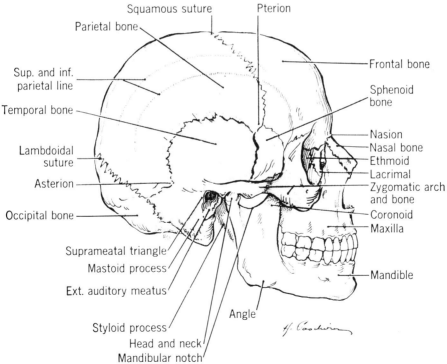

Squamous suture
Pterion
Parietal bone
Sup. and inf. parietal line
Temporal bone
Lambdoidal suture
Asterion
Occipital bone
Suprameatal triangle
Mastoid process
Ext. auditory meatus
Styloid process
Head and neck
Mandibular notch
Angle

Frontal bone
Sphenoid bone
Nasion
Nasal bone
Ethmoid
Lacrimal
Zygomatic arch and bone
Coronoid
Maxilla
Mandible

Plate 8. Norma of skull, anterior and lateral views. (Reprinted from *Stedman's Medical Dictionary*, Ed. 20. The Williams & Wilkins Co., Baltimore, 1961.)

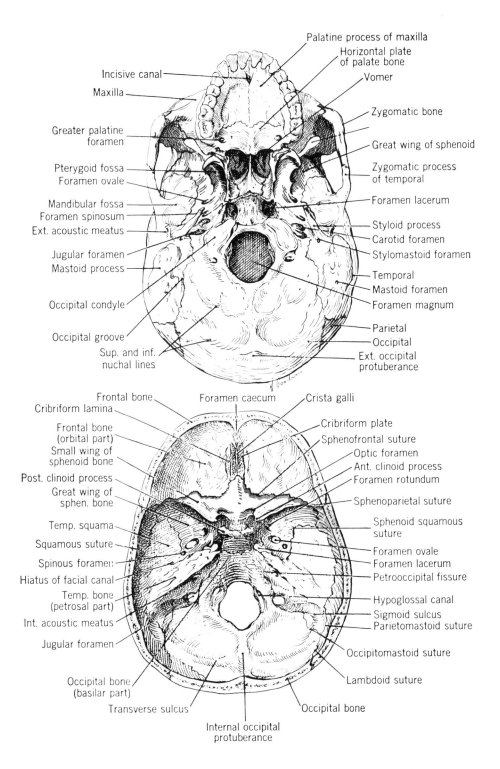

Plate 9. Norma of skull, top and bottom views. (Reprinted from *Stedman's Medical Dictionary*, Ed. 20. The Williams & Wilkins Co., Baltimore, 1961.)

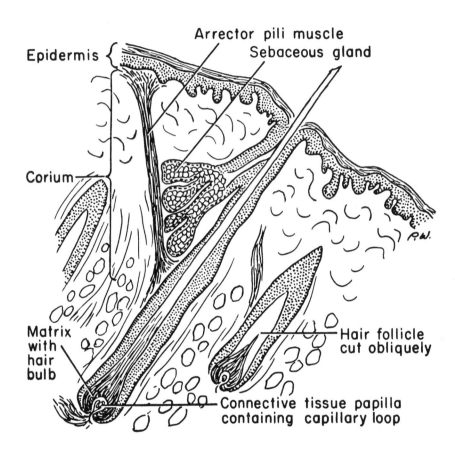

Epidermis {

Arrector pili muscle

Sebaceous gland

Corium

Matrix
with
hair
bulb

Hair follicle
cut obliquely

Connective tissue papilla
containing capillary loop

Plate 10. Structure of skin with longitudinal section of hair follicle.

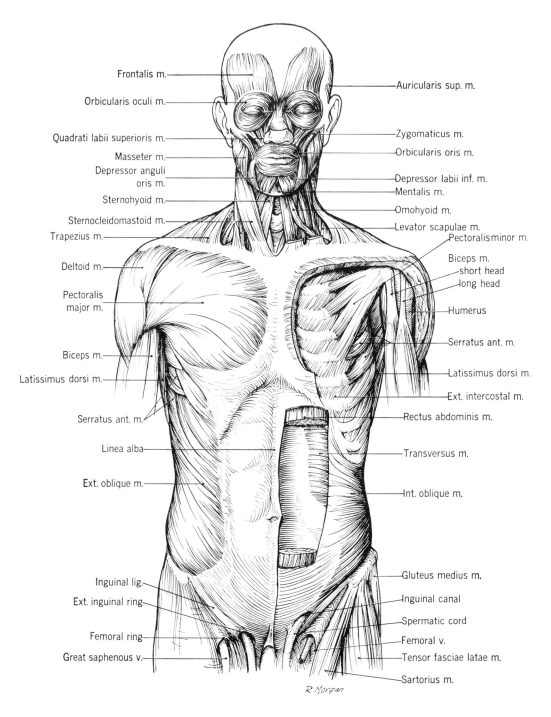

Frontalis m.

Orbicularis oculi m.

Quadrati labii superioris m.

Masseter m.

Depressor anguli oris m.

Sternohyoid m.

Sternocleidomastoid m.

Trapezius m.

Deltoid m.

Pectoralis major m.

Biceps m.

Latissimus dorsi m.

Serratus ant. m.

Linea alba

Ext. oblique m.

Inguinal lig.

Ext. inguinal ring

Femoral ring

Great saphenous v.

Auricularis sup. m.

Zygomaticus m.

Orbicularis oris m.

Depressor labii inf. m.

Mentalis m.

Omohyoid m.

Levator scapulae m.

Pectoralis minor m.

Biceps m.
short head
long head

Humerus

Serratus ant. m.

Latissimus dorsi m.

Ext. intercostal m.

Rectus abdominis m.

Transversus m.

Int. oblique m.

Gluteus medius m.

Inguinal canal

Spermatic cord

Femoral v.

Tensor fasciae latae m.

Sartorius m.

R. Morgan

Plate 11. Muscles of head, neck and torso, anterior view. (Reprinted from *Stedman's Medical Dictionary*, Ed. 20. The Williams & Wilkins Co., Baltimore, 1961.)

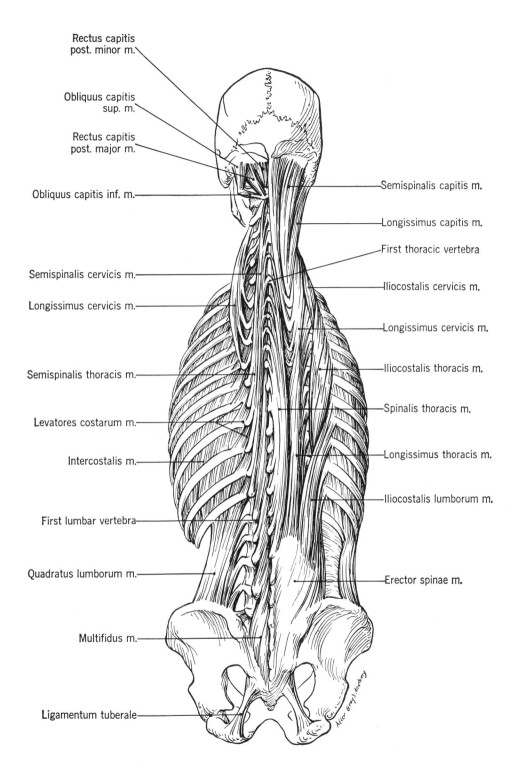

Rectus capitis
post. minor m.

Obliquus capitis
sup. m.

Rectus capitis
post. major m.

Obliquus capitis inf. m.

Semispinalis cervicis m.

Longissimus cervicis m.

Semispinalis thoracis m.

Levatores costarum m.

Intercostalis m.

First lumbar vertebra

Quadratus lumborum m.

Multifidus m.

Ligamentum tuberale

Semispinalis capitis m.

Longissimus capitis m.

First thoracic vertebra

Iliocostalis cervicis m.

Longissimus cervicis m.

Iliocostalis thoracis m.

Spinalis thoracis m.

Longissimus thoracis m.

Iliocostalis lumborum m.

Erector spinae m.

Plate 12. Muscles of back, deep dissection. (Reprinted from *Stedman's Medical Dictionary*, Ed. 20. The Williams & Wilkins Co., Baltimore, 1961.)

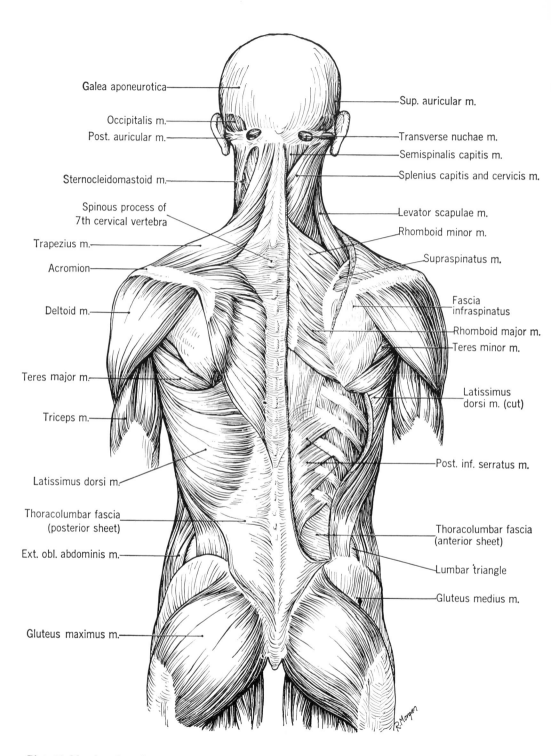

Galea aponeurotica

Occipitalis m.

Post. auricular m.

Sternocleidomastoid m.

Spinous process of
7th cervical vertebra

Trapezius m.

Acromion

Deltoid m.

Teres major m.

Triceps m.

Latissimus dorsi m.

Thoracolumbar fascia
(posterior sheet)

Ext. obl. abdominis m.

Gluteus maximus m.

Sup. auricular m.

Transverse nuchae m.

Semispinalis capitis m.

Splenius capitis and cervicis m.

Levator scapulae m.

Rhomboid minor m.

Supraspinatus m.

Fascia
infraspinatus

Rhomboid major m.

Teres minor m.

Latissimus
dorsi m. (cut)

Post. inf. serratus m.

Thoracolumbar fascia
(anterior sheet)

Lumbar triangle

Gluteus medius m.

Plate 13. Muscles of trunk, posterior view. (Reprinted from *Stedman's Medical Dictionary*, Ed. 20. The Williams & Wilkins Co., Baltimore, 1961.)

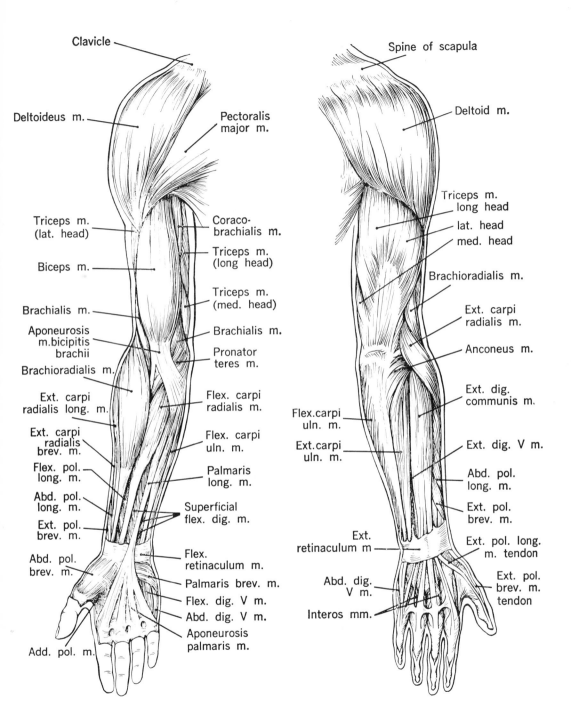

Clavicle

Deltoideus m.

Pectoralis
major m.

Spine of scapula

Deltoid m.

Triceps m.
(lat. head)

Coraco-
brachialis m.

Triceps m.
long head
lat. head
med. head

Biceps m.

Triceps m.
(long head)

Brachioradialis m.

Brachialis m.

Triceps m.
(med. head)

Aponeurosis
m.bicipitis
brachii

Brachialis m.

Ext. carpi
radialis m.

Brachioradialis m.

Pronator
teres m.

Anconeus m.

Ext. carpi
radialis long. m.

Flex. carpi
radialis m.

Ext. carpi
radialis
brev. m.

Flex. carpi
uln. m.

Flex.carpi
uln. m.

Ext. dig.
communis m.

Flex. pol.
long. m.

Palmaris
long. m.

Ext.carpi
uln. m.

Ext. dig. V m.

Abd. pol.
long. m.

Superficial
flex. dig. m.

Abd. pol.
long. m.

Ext. pol.
brev. m.

Ext. pol.
brev. m.

Ext. pol.
brev. m.

Abd. pol.
brev. m.

Flex.
retinaculum m.

Ext.
retinaculum m

Ext. pol. long.
m. tendon

Palmaris brev. m.

Abd. dig.
V m.

Ext. pol.
brev. m.
tendon

Flex. dig. V m.

Abd. dig. V m.

Interos mm.

Add. pol. m.

Aponeurosis
palmaris m.

Plate 14. Superficial muscles of right upper extremity. (Reprinted from *Stedman's Medical Dictionary*, Ed. 20. The Williams & Wilkins Co., Baltimore, 1961.)

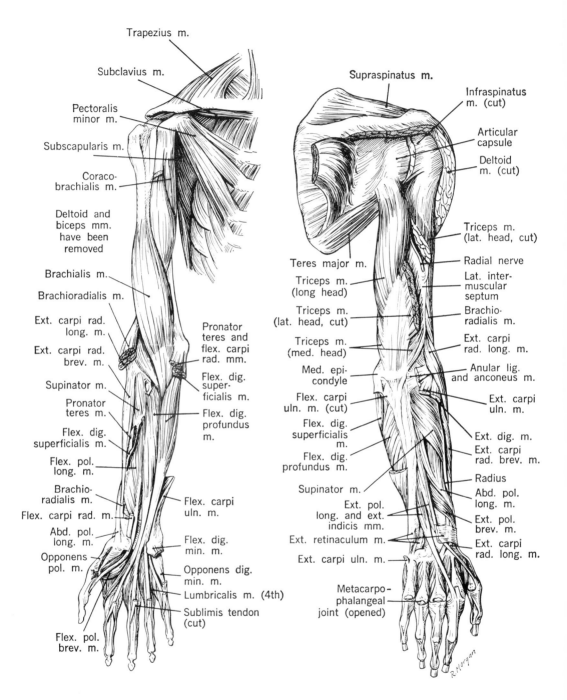

Plate 15. Muscles of right upper extremity, deep dissection. (Reprinted from *Stedman's Medical Dictionary*, Ed. 20. The Williams & Wilkins Co., Baltimore, 1961.)

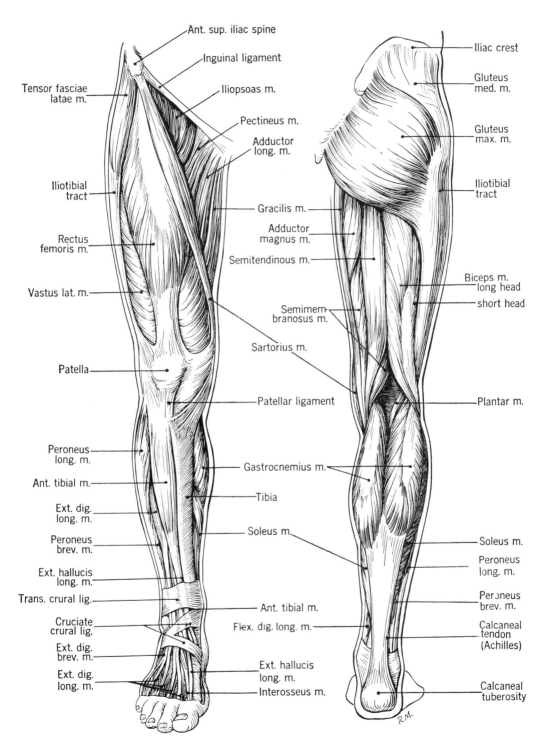

Ant. sup. iliac spine

Inguinal ligament

Iliac crest

Tensor fasciae latae m.

Iliopsoas m.

Gluteus med. m.

Pectineus m.

Adductor long. m.

Gluteus max. m.

Iliotibial tract

Iliotibial tract

Rectus femoris m.

Gracilis m.

Adductor magnus m.

Semitendinous m.

Biceps m. long head

short head

Vastus lat. m.

Semimembranosus m.

Sartorius m.

Patella

Patellar ligament

Plantar m.

Peroneus long. m.

Gastrocnemius m.

Ant. tibial m.

Tibia

Ext. dig. long. m.

Soleus m.

Peroneus brev. m.

Soleus m.

Ext. hallucis long. m.

Peroneus long. m.

Trans. crural lig.

Ant. tibial m.

Peroneus brev. m.

Cruciate crural lig.

Flex. dig. long. m.

Calcaneal tendon (Achilles)

Ext. dig. brev. m.

Ext. hallucis long. m.

Ext. dig. long. m.

Interosseus m.

Calcaneal tuberosity

R.M.

Plate 16. Superficial muscles of right lower extremity. (Reprinted from *Stedman's Medical Dictionary*, Ed. 20. The Williams & Wilkins Co., Baltimore, 1961.)

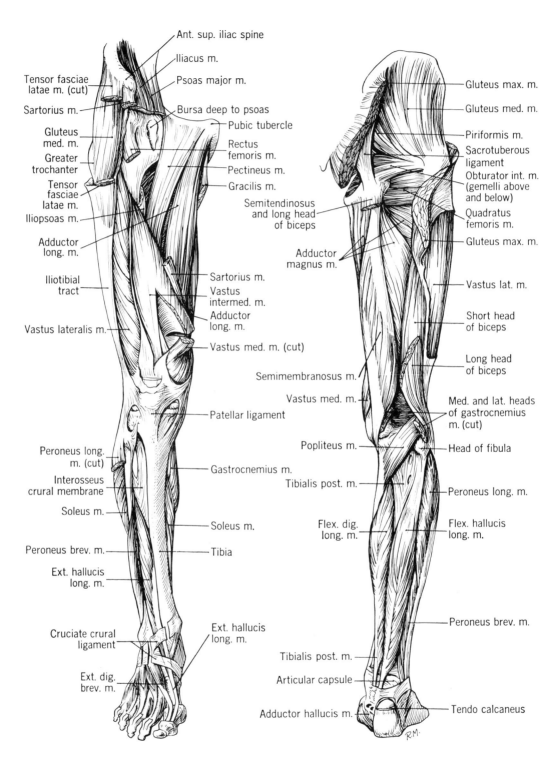

Plate 17. Muscles of right lower extremity, deep dissection. (Reprinted from *Stedman's Medical Diction-ary*, Ed. 20. The Williams & Wilkins Co., Baltimore, 1961.)

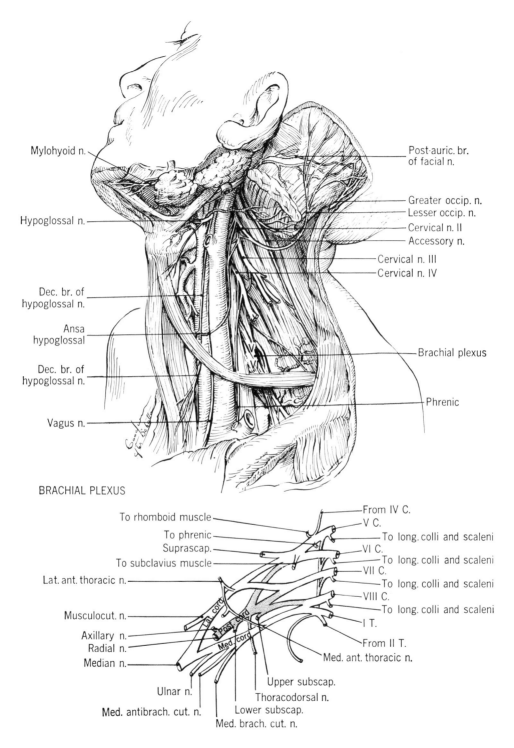

BRACHIAL PLEXUS

Plate 18. Nerves of neck and axilla. (Reprinted from *Stedman's Medical Dictionary*, Ed. 20. The Williams & Wilkins Co., Baltimore, 1961.)

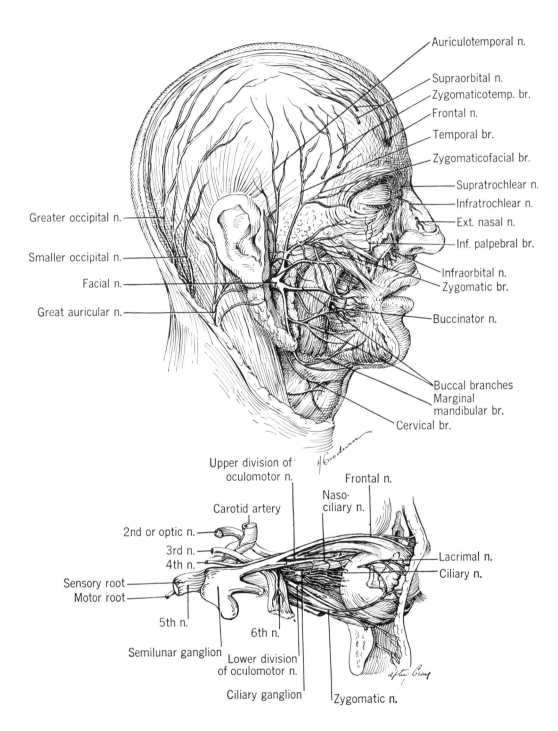

Auriculotemporal n.

Supraorbital n.
Zygomaticotemp. br.
Frontal n.
Temporal br.
Zygomaticofacial br.
Supratrochlear n.
Infratrochlear n.
Ext. nasal n.
Inf. palpebral br.
Infraorbital n.
Zygomatic br.
Buccinator n.

Greater occipital n.

Smaller occipital n.
Facial n.
Great auricular n.

Buccal branches
Marginal
mandibular br.
Cervical br.

Upper division of
oculomotor n.
Frontal n.
Naso-
ciliary n.
Carotid artery
2nd or optic n.
3rd n.
4th n.
Lacrimal n.
Ciliary n.
Sensory root
Motor root
5th n.
6th n.
Semilunar ganglion
Lower division
of oculomotor n.
Ciliary ganglion
Zygomatic n.

Plate 19. Nerves of orbit and maxillary region. (Reprinted from *Stedman's Medical Dictionary*. Ed. 20 The Williams & Wilkins Co., Baltimore, 1961.)

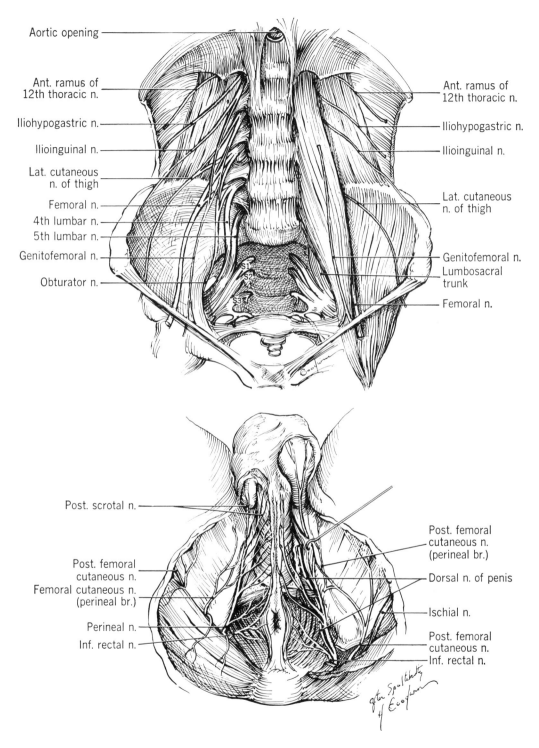

Aortic opening

Ant. ramus of
12th thoracic n.

Iliohypogastric n.

Ilioinguinal n.

Lat. cutaneous
n. of thigh

Femoral n.

4th lumbar n.

5th lumbar n.

Genitofemoral n.

Obturator n.

Ant. ramus of
12th thoracic n.

Iliohypogastric n.

Ilioinguinal n.

Lat. cutaneous
n. of thigh

Genitofemoral n.

Lumbosacral
trunk

Femoral n.

Post. scrotal n.

Post. femoral
cutaneous n.
(perineal br.)

Dorsal n. of penis

Post. femoral
cutaneous n.
Femoral cutaneous n.
(perineal br.)

Ischial n.

Perineal n.

Inf. rectal n.

Post. femoral
cutaneous n.

Inf. rectal n.

Plate 20. Nerves of lumbar plexus. (Reprinted from *Stedman's Medical Dictionary*, Ed. 20. The Williams & Wilkins Co., Baltimore, 1961.)

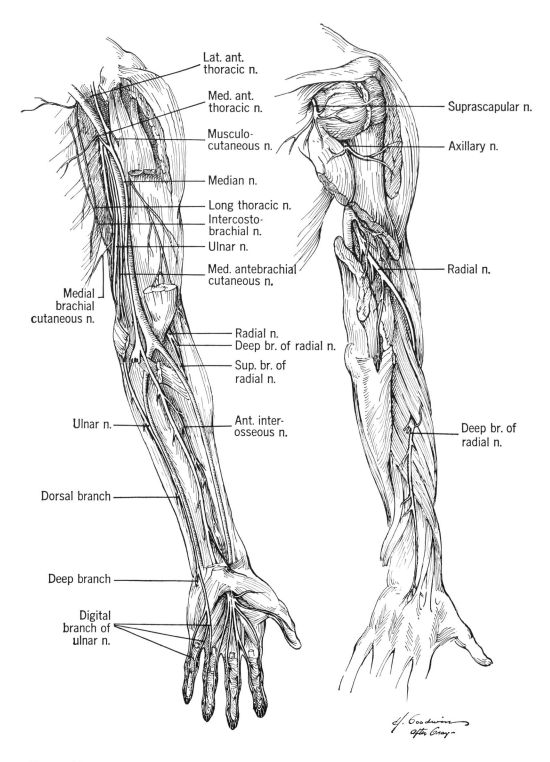

Lat. ant.
thoracic n.

Med. ant.
thoracic n.

Musculo-
cutaneous n.

Median n.

Long thoracic n.

Intercosto-
brachial n.

Ulnar n.

Med. antebrachial
cutaneous n.

Medial
brachial
cutaneous n.

Radial n.

Deep br. of radial n.

Sup. br. of
radial n.

Ulnar n.

Ant. inter-
osseous n.

Dorsal branch

Deep branch

Digital
branch of
ulnar n.

Suprascapular n.

Axillary n.

Radial n.

Deep br. of
radial n.

Plate 21. Nerves of upper extremity. (Reprinted from *Stedman's Medical Dictionary*, Ed. 20. The Williams & Wilkins Co., Baltimore, 1961.)

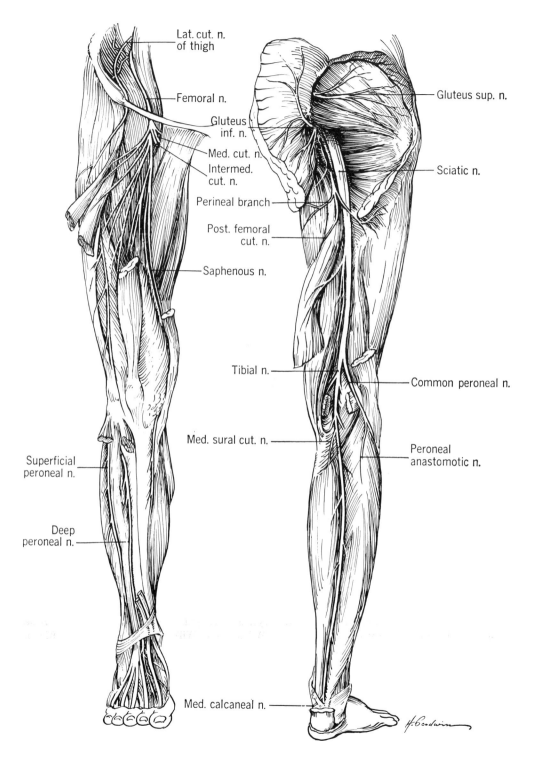

Lat. cut. n.
of thigh

Femoral n.

Gluteus
inf. n.

Med. cut. n.
Intermed.
cut. n.

Perineal branch

Post. femoral
cut. n.

Saphenous n.

Tibial n.

Med. sural cut. n.

Superficial
peroneal n.

Deep
peroneal n.

Med. calcaneal n.

Gluteus sup. n.

Sciatic n.

Common peroneal n.

Peroneal
anastomotic n.

H. Goodwin

Plate 22. Nerves of lower extremity, anterior and posterior views. (Reprinted from *Stedman's Medical Dictionary*, Ed. 20. The Williams & Wilkins Co., Baltimore, 1961.)

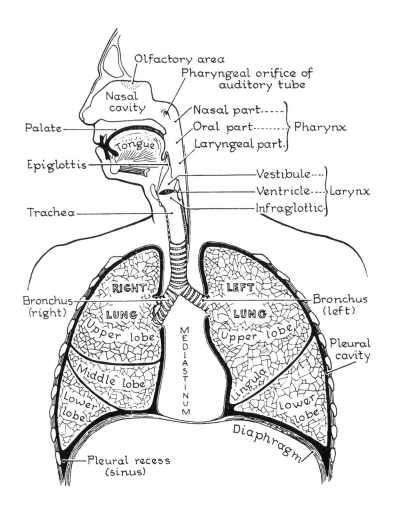

Plate 23. Diagram of the respiratory system. (Reprinted from Grant, J. C. Boileau, and Basmajian, J. V.: *Method of Anatomy*, Ed. 7. The Williams & Wilkins Co., Baltimore, 1965, p. 55.)

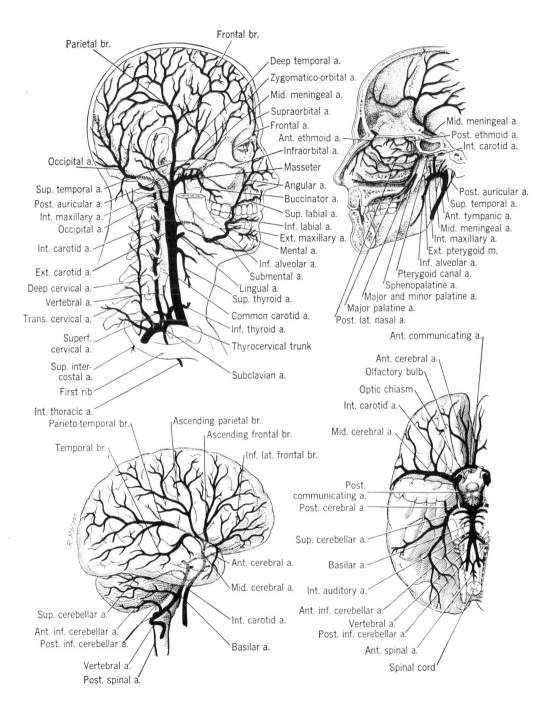

Plate 24. Arteries of head and brain. (Reprinted from *Stedman's Medical Dictionary*, Ed. 20. The Williams & Wilkins Co., Baltimore, 1961.)

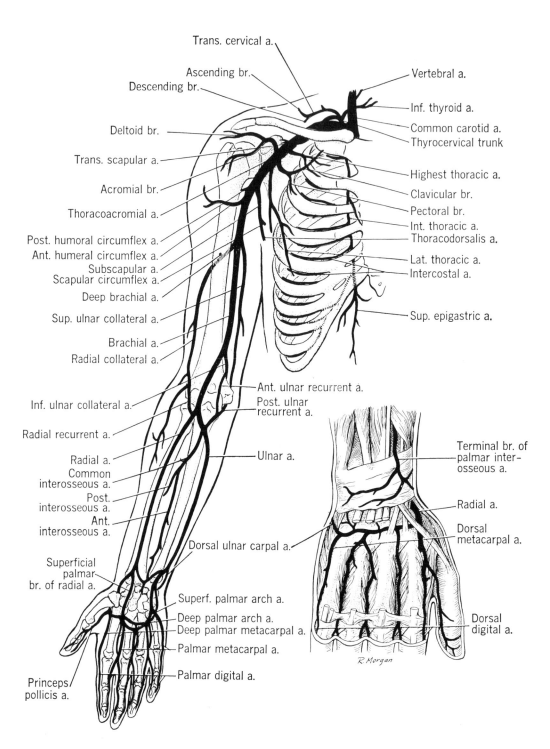

Plate 25. Arteries of upper extremity and chest. (Reprinted from *Stedman's Medical Dictionary*, Ed. 20. The Williams & Wilkins Co., Baltimore, 1961.)

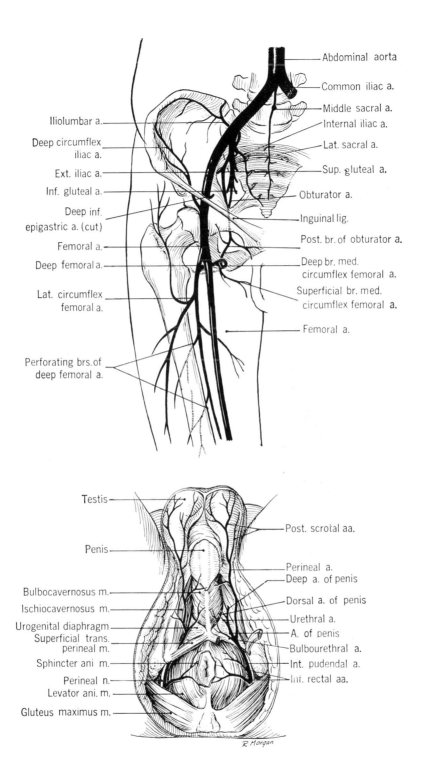

Abdominal aorta

Common iliac a.

Middle sacral a.

Internal iliac a.

Lat. sacral a.

Sup. gluteal a.

Obturator a.

Inguinal lig.

Post. br. of obturator a.

Deep br. med.
circumflex femoral a.

Superficial br. med.
circumflex femoral a.

Femoral a.

Iliolumbar a.

Deep circumflex
iliac a.

Ext. iliac a.

Inf. gluteal a.

Deep inf.
epigastric a. (cut)

Femoral a.

Deep femoral a.

Lat. circumflex
femoral a.

Perforating brs. of
deep femoral a.

Testis

Penis

Bulbocavernosus m.

Ischiocavernosus m.

Urogenital diaphragm

Superficial trans.
perineal m.

Sphincter ani m.

Perineal n.

Levator ani. m.

Gluteus maximus m.

Post. scrotal aa.

Perineal a.

Deep a. of penis

Dorsal a. of penis

Urethral a.

A. of penis

Bulbourethral a.

Int. pudendal a.

Inf. rectal aa.

R Morgan

Plate 26. Arteries of thigh and perineum. (Reprinted from *Stedman's Medical Dictionary*, Ed. 20. The Williams & Wilkins Co., Baltimore, 1961.)

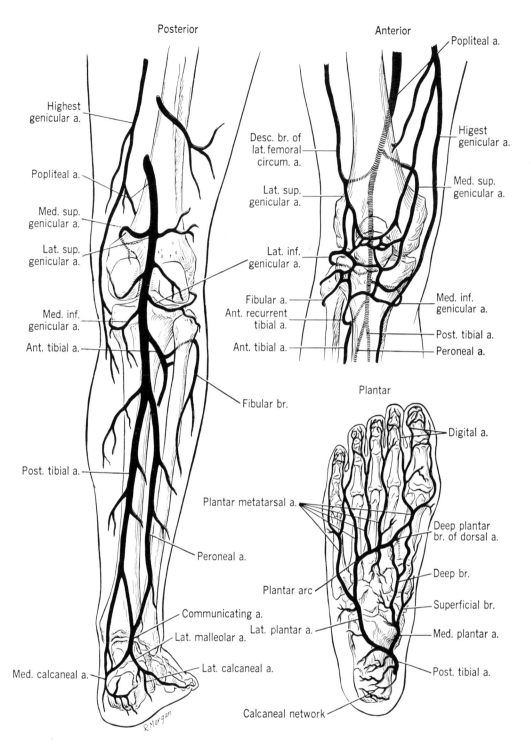

Plate 27. Arteries of right lower extremity in relation to bones. (Reprinted from *Stedman's Medical Dictionary,* Ed. 20. The Williams & Wilkins Co., Baltimore, 1961.)

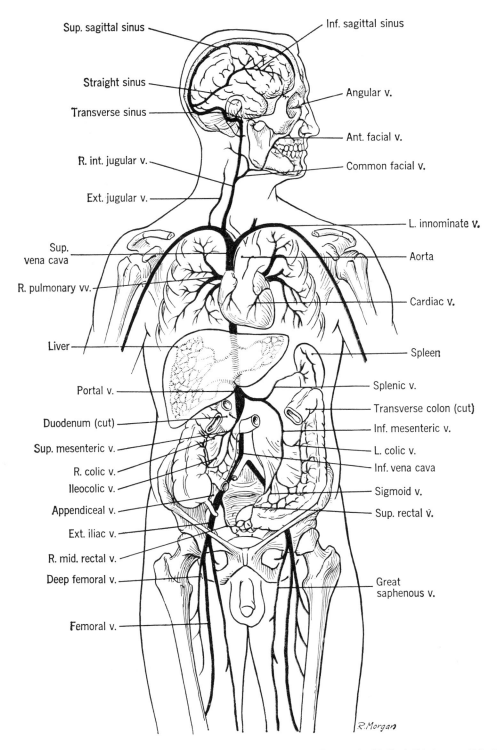

Sup. sagittal sinus

Inf. sagittal sinus

Straight sinus

Angular v.

Transverse sinus

Ant. facial v.

R. int. jugular v.

Common facial v.

Ext. jugular v.

L. innominate v.

Sup.
vena cava

Aorta

R. pulmonary vv.

Cardiac v.

Liver

Spleen

Portal v.

Splenic v.

Duodenum (cut)

Transverse colon (cut)

Inf. mesenteric v.

Sup. mesenteric v.

L. colic v.

R. colic v.

Inf. vena cava

Ileocolic v.

Sigmoid v.

Appendiceal v.

Sup. rectal v.

Ext. iliac v.

R. mid. rectal v.

Deep femoral v.

Great
saphenous v.

Femoral v.

R. Morgan

Plate 28. Veins, anterior view, viscera exposed. (Reprinted from *Stedman's Medical Dictionary*, Ed. 20.
The Williams & Wilkins Co., Baltimore, 1961.)

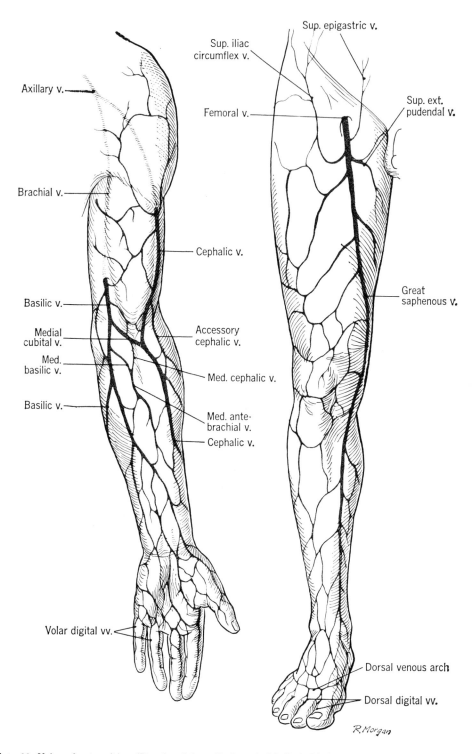

Plate 29. Veins of extremities. (Reprinted from *Stedman's Medical Dictionary*, Ed. 20. The Williams & Wilkins Co., Baltimore, 1961.)

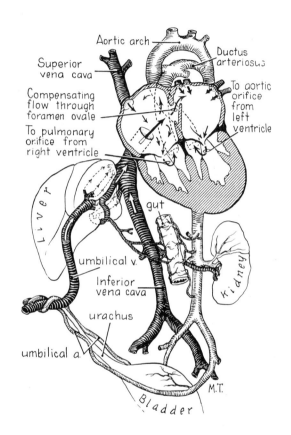

Plate 30. Fetal circulation. (Reprinted from *Stedman's Medical Dictionary*, Ed. 20. The Williams & Wilkins Co., Baltimore, 1961, p. 572.)

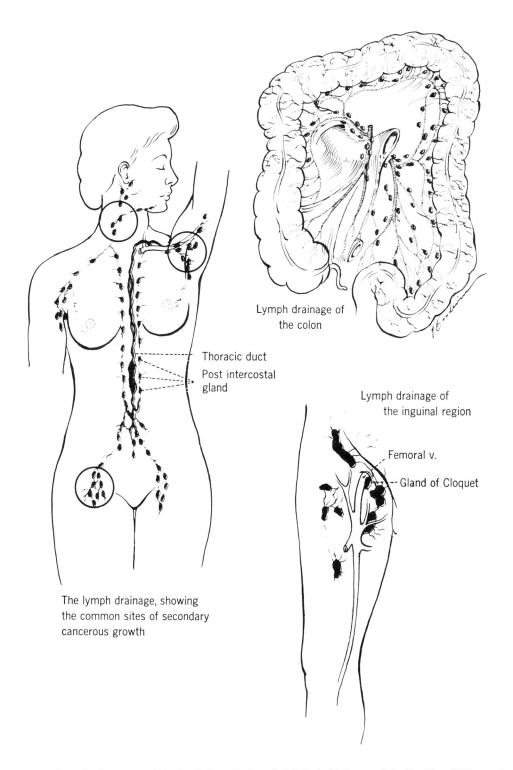

Lymph drainage of
the colon

Thoracic duct

Post intercostal
gland

Lymph drainage of
the inguinal region

Femoral v.

-- Gland of Cloquet

The lymph drainage, showing
the common sites of secondary
cancerous growth

Plate 31. Lymphatic system. (Reprinted from *Stedman's Medical Dictionary*, Ed. 20. The Williams & Wilkins Co., Baltimore, 1961.)

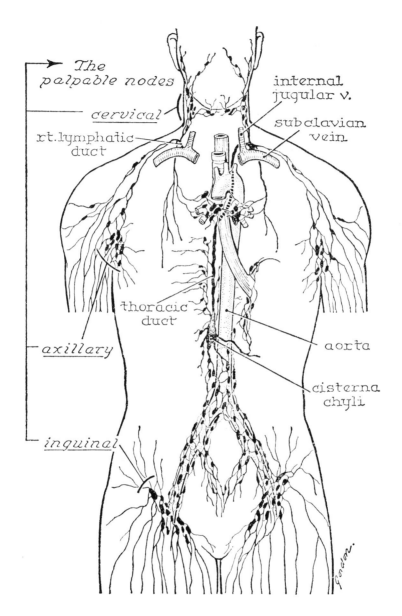

Plate 32. Scheme of lymphatic system. (Reprinted from Basmajian, J. V.: *Primary Anatomy*, Ed. 5. The Williams & Wilkins Co., Baltimore, 1961, p. 289.)

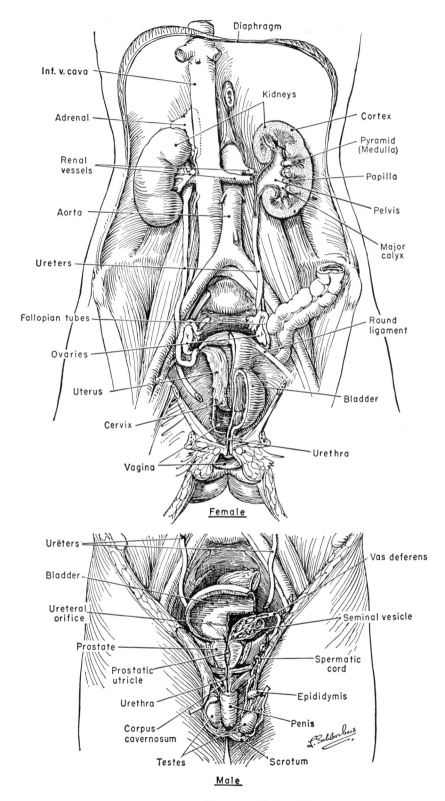

Plate 33. Urogenital system. From *Dorland's Illustrated Medical Dictionary*, Ed. 23. W. B. Saunders Co., Philadelphia, 1958, p. 1356. Reprinted with the permission of the W. B. Saunders Co.)

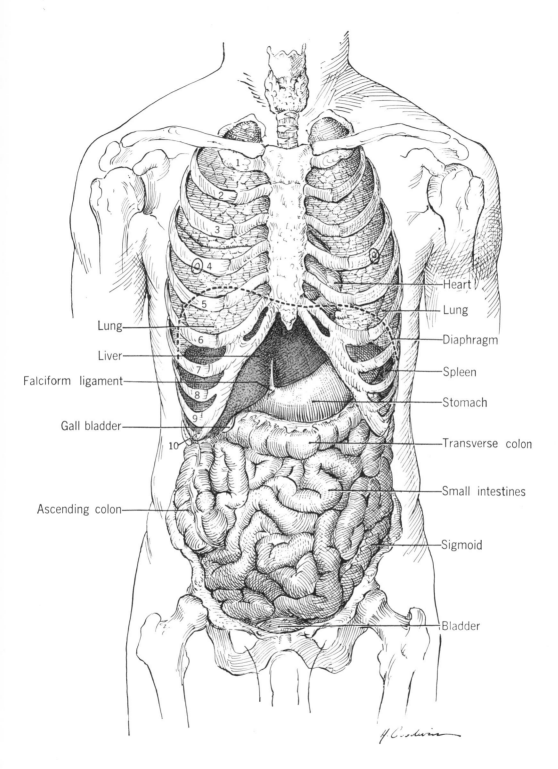

Lung

Liver

Falciform ligament

Gall bladder

Ascending colon

Heart

Lung

Diaphragm

Spleen

Stomach

Transverse colon

Small intestines

Sigmoid

Bladder

Plate 34. Abdominal and thoracic viscera, anterior view (after Pernkopf). (Reprinted from *Stedman's Medical Dictionary*, Ed. 20. The Williams & Wilkins Co., Baltimore, 1961.)

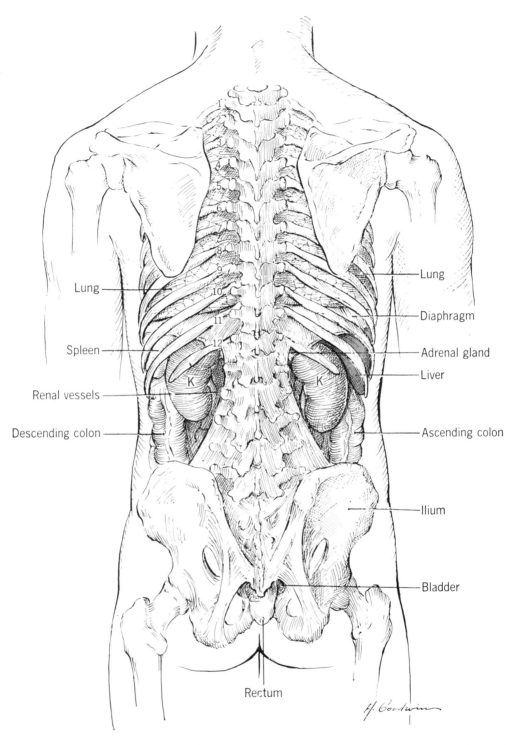

Plate 35. Abdominal and thoracic viscera, posterior view (after Pernkopf). (Reprinted from *Stedman's Medical Dictionary*, Ed. 20. The Williams & Wilkins Co., Baltimore, 1961.)

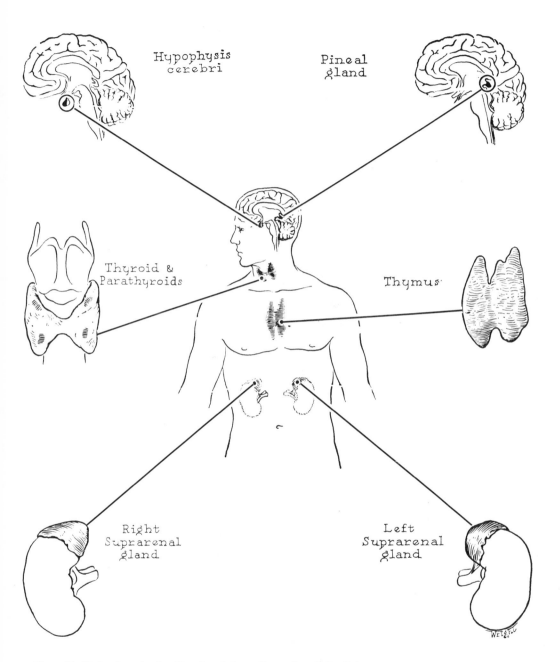

Plate 36. Endocrine glands. (Reprinted from Basmajian, J. V.: *Primary Anatomy*, Ed. 5. The Williams & Wilkins Co., Baltimore, 1964, p. 355.)

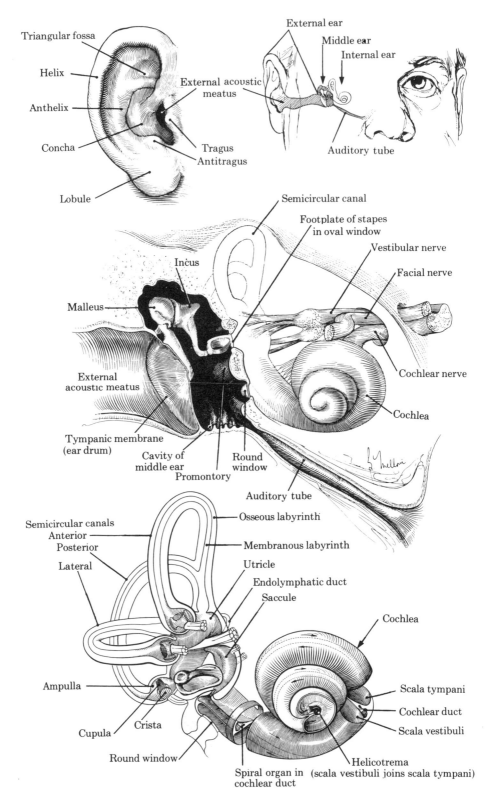

Plate 37. External and internal structure of ear. (From *Dorland's Illustrated Medical Dictionary*, Ed. 24. W. B. Saunders Co., Philadelphia, 1965. Reprinted with the permission of the W. B. Saunders Co.)

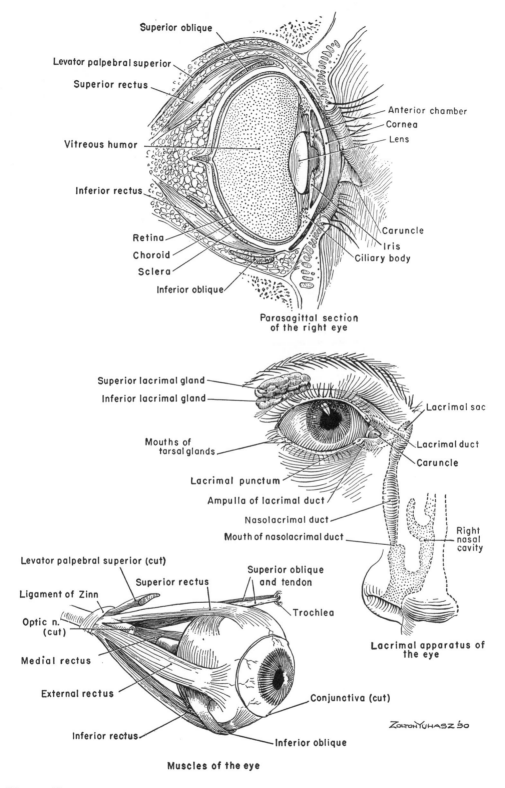

Superior oblique

Levator palpebral superior

Superior rectus

Vitreous humor

Inferior rectus

Retina

Choroid

Sclera

Inferior oblique

Anterior chamber

Cornea

Lens

Caruncle

Iris

Ciliary body

Parasagittal section
of the right eye

Superior lacrimal gland

Inferior lacrimal gland

**Mouths of
tarsal glands**

Lacrimal punctum

Ampulla of lacrimal duct

Nasolacrimal duct

Mouth of nasolacrimal duct

Lacrimal sac

Lacrimal duct

Caruncle

Right
nasal
cavity

Lacrimal apparatus of
the eye

Levator palpebral superior (cut)

Superior rectus

Ligament of Zinn

**Optic n.
(cut)**

Medial rectus

External rectus

Inferior rectus

**Superior oblique
and tendon**

Trochlea

Conjunctiva (cut)

Inferior oblique

ZOLTONYUHASZ 50

Muscles of the eye

Plate 38. The eye and related structures. (From *Dorland's Illustrated Medical Dictionary*, Ed. 23. W. B. Saunders Co., Philadelphia, 1958. Reprinted with the permission of the W. B. Saunders Co.)

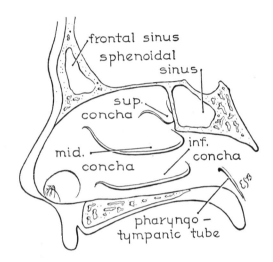

frontal sinus
sphenoidal sinus
sup. concha
inf. concha
mid. concha
pharyngo–tympanic tube

Plate 39. Lateral wall of nose. (Reprinted from Basmajian, J. V.: *Primary Anatomy*, Ed. 5. The Williams & Wilkins Co., Baltimore, 1964.)

SURGICAL PROCEDURES— NERVOUS SYSTEM

Cranium (The Skull or Brain Pan)
Incision

Craniotomy: Any operation on the cranium such as trephine for tumor, aneurysm. AV malformation, cicatrix excision, depressed fracture, gunshot wound, subdural hematoma, epidural hematoma, intracerebral hematoma, hypophysectomy, thalamotomy and for cranial bony abnormalities.

Encephalotomy: The operation for destroying the brain of a fetus to facilitate delivery; also, dissection of the brain.

Excision

Craniectomy: Excision of a part of the skull.

Linear craniectomy: (Parasagittal, coronal, or lambdoid): Excision of a strip of the skull for relief of craniostenosis.

Chordotomy: Dissection of any cord to relieve pain.

Cingulectomy: Extirpation of the anterior half of the gyrus cinguli (bilateral).

Repair

Cranioplasty: Plastic operation on the skull with bone graft or insertion of metal or plastic plate.

Repair of an encephalocele: A protrusion of the brain through a cranial fissure.

Repair of a meningocele (spina bifida): A congenital hernia in which the meninges protrude through an opening of the skull or spinal column. In spina bifida, a congenital defect in wall of the spinal canal caused by lack of union between laminae of the vertebrae.

Open reduction of fracture of skull, with elevation or removal of fragments; debridement of compound fracture of skull.

Incision

Drainage of subdural, epidural or subarachnoid spaces for abscess or hematoma, cranial or spinal.

Lumbar puncture: Puncture [rachiocentesis] of the lumbar subarachnoid space to secure spinal fluid and measure intracranial pressure for analysis.

Excision

Ventriculotomy: Puncture of a cerebral ventricle.

Brain
Incision

Frontal lobotomy (unilateral or bilateral by craniotomy): A bilateral small trephination in the plane of the coronal suture through which the white matter of the brain is sectioned. Thus disconnecting the diencephalon, especially the hypothalmic area from the prefrontal cortex by section of the white fiber connecting pathways subcortically in a plane that passes adjacent to the anterior tip of the lateral ventricle and posterior margin of the sphenoid wing for relief of mental disturbances.

Excision

Excision of a cortical scar.

Excision of brain cyst, neoplasm or abscess.

Topectomy: Excision of the cerebral lobe or lobes.

Introduction

Injection of alcohol (intraspinal, paravertebral or paracranial).

Injection of alcohol (second and third divisons for trigeminal neuralgia).

OTHER NEUROSURGICAL PROCEDURES

Stereotactic Procedures
Stereotaxy: A method of inserting instruments into precise areas of the brain through small openings in the skull by means of a stereotaxic instrument.

Stereoencephalotomy: Production of sharply circumscribed lesions in subcortical ganglia or pathways by means of electrodes whose direction and position in space is determined by mechanical guides so as to avoid as far as possible unintended lesions in other areas.

Thalamotomy: Production of circumscribed lesions in the thalamus, anterior nucleus of the thalamus, or in the dorsomedial nucleus of the thalamus.

Pallidotomy: Surgical section of nerve fibers coming from the globus pallidus to produce changes in pathological involuntary movements in man.

Decompressions

Subtemporal decompression: Removal of pressure, usually in the subtemporal, or lateral region of the head above the zygoma.

Cerebral decompression: Removal of a flap of the skull and incision of the dura mater for the purpose of relieving intracranial pressure.

Transfrontal Orbitotomy: Exposure of the orbital margin to decompress its roof and for exploration and remove when possible neoplasms in the suborbital region.

Shunts

Ventriculocisternostomy: Establishment of a communication between the ventricle cistern and the cisterna magna (an intracranial shunt) (a Torkildsen procedure).

Ventriculoatriostomy (VA): A shunt channeling cerebrospinal fluid from the lateral ventricle through the subcutaneous tissues and jugular vein into the right atrium of the heart.

Ventriculomastoidostomy: An establishment of a communication in which the lateral cerebral ventricle is connected to the mastoid antrum.

Subarachnoidureterostomy: A shunt to establish communication between the subarachnoid space of the lumbar spine through the deep back muscles into one of the ureters.

Nerve Block

Paravertebral block, lumbar or thoracic.

Sympathetic block (cervical).

Stellate ganglion.

Brachial plexus block.

Intercostal nerves.

Lumbar, sacral and coccygeal nerves.

Pudendal nerve.

Splanchnic nerves

Ilioinguinal and iliohypogastric nerves.

Sciatic nerve.

Phrenic nerve.

Other peripheral nerves.

Destruction

Neurolysis: Surgical breaking up of perineural adhesions.

Destruction or dissolution of nerve tissue.

Repair

Neuroplasty: Plastic repair of nerve injuries.

Neuroanastomosis: Operation of forming an anastomosis of nerves.

Neurectasy, neurectasia, neurectasis: Surgical nerve stretching.

Autonomic Nervous System

Excision

Sympathectomy: Surgical transection, resection, or other interruption of some portion of the sympathetic nervous system.

Spinal Cord and Nerve Roots

Incision

Tractotomy: Operation of severing or incising a nerve tract.

Chordotomy: Surgical division of the anterolateral tracts of the spinal cord (for intractable pain).

Rachiotomy: Surgical opening of spinal canal.

Rachitomy: Cutting of vertebral column in surgery or in obstetrics.

Rhizotomy (also radicotomy): Division or transection of nerve roots.

Laminotomy: Dividing the lamina of a vertebra.

Excision

Foraminotomy: Surgical removal of the roof of the intervertebral foramina for relief of a nerve root compression.

Laminectomy: Excision of the posterior arch of a vertebra.

Radiculectomy: Resection of spinal nerve roots.

Mesencephalotomy: Sectioning of structures in the midbrain primarily for relief of intractable pain.

Peripheral Nerves, Cerebral Nerves and Ganglia

Incision

Neurotomy: A surgical cutting, division or transection of a nerve, or nerve.

Retrogasserian neurotomy: Transection of the sensory root of the gasserian ganglion.

Phrenicotomy: Surgical division of the phrenic nerve and its accessory; transection of the trigeminal and the glossopharyngeal nerves.

Transection: Spinal nerves, of occipital nerve, or of 8th cranial nerve for Meniere's syndrome.

Excision

Phrenicectomy (phrenicexairesis): Resection of a part of the phrenic nerve.

Neurexeresis: Avulsion of a nerve to relieve neuralgia.

Neurectomy: Partial or total excision or resection of a nerve (unilateral or bilateral).

Splanchnicotomy: Surgical section of a splanchnic nerve.

Splanchniectomy: Also combined with sympathectomy for the relief of hypertension.

Excision of a section of the greater splanchnic nerve.

Repair

Neuroanastomosis: The operation of forming an anastomosis of nerves.

Neurectasy, neurectasia and neurectasis: Surgical nerve stretching.

Ulnar nerve transposition: for delayed ulnar palsy.

RESPIRATORY SYSTEM

Now set the teeth and stretch the nostril wide, Hold hard the breath and bend up every spirit to his full height. HENRY V; SHAKESPEARE

The organs of breathing consist of a series of air passages including the (nasal chambers), pharynx, larynx, trachea and bronchi, and the lungs, to which these passages lead (Plate 23). The mouth serves as a secondary respiratory passage, if the nasal passages are blocked. In man, the pharynx is a pathway used both by the digestive and respiratory system. The pharynx is therefore included as part of the digestive system. The nose possesses an area specialized to register the sense of smell, and is therefore referred to with the sensory system. However, it does serve as a passageway of air going to and from the lungs.

Respiration is breathing, a function consisting of supplying oxygen to all of the cells of the body and the removal of the products of oxidation in the tissues, mainly carbon dioxide from them. While we are only rarely conscious of breathing, which continues rhythmically without voluntary effort on our part, holding one's breath for a limited time would be an example of some voluntary control of this vital process.

The exchange of gases is known as respiration, at two sites: the exchange across the respiratory membrane with the blood in the capillaries of the pulmonary circulation is called external respiration; diffusion of gases between the systemic capillaries and the cells is called internal respiration.

Accessory functions of the respiratory system are coughing and sneezing, which are protective; talking, which makes possible the communication of ideas; and finally, the sensation of smell which is dependent upon the respiratory system. The nasal cavity accessory functions are phonation, acting as a sounding board for the voice and in olfaction (smell).

The *larynx* (voice box) comprises exquisitely fashioned and delicately poised cartilages and cords, placed at the upper part of the air passage and situated between the trachea and the root of the tongue, and moved by especially sensitive muscles. A sphincter valve, the epiglottis, is on duty at the entrance to the windpipe, preventing food from entering the larynx controlling the air flow, and at times closing the valve so that thoracic pressure may be raised to clear the upper airway by expulsive effort when the valve is suddenly opened. But it is not specialized for speech. The cartilages of the larynx are the thyroid, cricoid and epiglottic, and the right and left arytenoids, corniculates and cuneiforms.

The *trachea* or windpipe is a flexible and expansile fibromuscular cylindrical tube approximately 4 inches long (11 centimeters) and 1 inch wide, beginning at the lower end of the larynx and passing into the thorax, terminates by dividing into the right and left bronchi, one for each lung, at the level of the upper border of the 5th thoracic vertebra and the sternal angle-junction between the manubrium and body of the sternum. The trachea is strengthened by 16 to 20 cartilages, sometimes referred to as "rings," horseshoe-shaped and opening posteriorly.

Bronchi and Bronchial Tree

The main bronchi are the two tubes into which the trachea divides, the right is shorter, wider, and more vertical than the left. They enter the right and left lung, respectively, and then break up into a great number of smaller branches, which are called bronchioles, less than one mm in diameter and having no cartilage in their walls.

Each bronchiole terminates in alveolar ducts and clusters of alveoli. Each bears on all parts of its surface small irregular projections known as alveloi, or air cells, which forms a lobule or unit of the lung tissue. Through these walls the blood is oxygenated.

Thoracic Cavity

Around the trachea, esophagus and blood vessels, the thoracic cavity is closed above in the root of the neck by a sheet of fascia (Sibson's fascia). Below, it is separated from the abdominal cavity by a sheet of muscle called the diaphragm. The thoracic cavity lodges the two pleural cavities, each containing a lung.

Lungs

The lungs are cone-shaped organs that lie in the pleural cavities of the thorax. The interpleural space between the two lungs is called the mediastinum, extending from the sternum in front to the thoracic vertebrae behind, and from the thoracic inlet above to the diaphragm below.

The interpleural space, the mediastinum, which separates the right and left lung, contains the heart, the great vessels, the thymus gland, the esophagus, certain nerves, a portion of the trachea and the principal bronchi.

The right lung is larger than the left, owing to the inclination of the heart to the left side, and is also shorter by one inch because of the diaphragm rising higher on the right side to accommodate the liver. It is divided by two interlobar fissures into superior, middle and inferior lobes. The left lung is smaller, and longer than the right lung and is divided into two lobes, the superior and inferior lobes.

SURGICAL PROCEDURES— RESPIRATORY SYSTEM

Accessory Sinuses: Frontal, Maxillary, Sphenoid and Ethmoid

Incision
> Ethmoidotomy: Surgical incision into the ethmoid sinus. Radical incision, (Caldwell-Luc) unilateral.
> Sinusotomy: Incision into a sinus: sphenoid, or frontal.

Excision
> Ethmoidectomy: Excision of the ethmoid cells, or a portion of the ethmoid bone.

Suture
> Closure of dental fistula of maxillary sinus with flap or radical antrotomy, (surgical opening of an antrum).
> Closure of an oro-nasal fistula (local mucoperiosteal pedicle flaps).

Larynx

Incision
> Laryngofissure: Operation of the larynx by a median incision through the thyroid cartilage for removal of a tumor.
> Laryngotomy: Surgical incision of the larynx.
> Thyrofissure: Surgical creation of an opening through the thyroid cartilage to gain access to interior of the larynx.

Excision
> Laryngopharyngectomy: Excision of the larynx and pharynx.
> Laryngectomy: Extirpation of the larynx.
> Hemilaryngectomy: Excision of one half of larynx.
> Epiglottidectomy: Excision of the epiglottis.

Suture
> Laryngorrhaphy: Suturing of the larynx.

Repair

Laryngoplasty: Plastic surgery of the larynx.

Introduction

Injection of radiopaque substance into larynx for bronchography; indirect method, or direct with bronchoscope.

Endoscopy

Laryngoscopy: Examination of the interior of the larynx by means of the laryngoscope.

Trachea and Bronchi

Incision

Tracheolaryngotomy: Incision of the trachea and larynx.

Tracheotomy: Formation of an artificial opening into the trachea.

Tracheostomy: Surgical formation of an opening into the trachea.

Suture

Tracheorrhaphy: Suturing the trachea.

Repair

Tracheoplasty: Plastic operations on the trachea.

Endoscopy

Bronchoscopy: Diagnostic, with biopsy, removal of a foreign body, excision of a tumor, aspiration of bronchus, drainage of lung abscess or cavity, and with lipiodol injection.

Bronchospirometry and catheterization of bronchi.

Tracheal aspiration under direct or indirect vision.

Repair

Bronchoplasty: Plastic surgery of the bronchus.

Lungs and Pleura

Incision

Thoracectomy: Thoracotomy with resection of a portion of a rib.

Thoracotomy: Surgical incision of the wall of the chest.

Thoracolaparotomy: Surgical incision through the thorax and abdomen.

Pneumonotomy: Surgical incision of a lung.

Thoracostomy: Surgical formation of an opening in the wall of the chest for the purpose of drainage.

Pleuracotomy: Surgical formation of an opening into a pleural cavity for evacuation or drainage.

Lobostomy: Surgical formation of an opening for performing external drainage of a lobe of the lung.

Pneumocentesis: Surgical puncture of lung for aspiration biopsy.

Thoracentesis: Surgical puncture of pleural cavity for aspiration.

Excision

Pneumectomy: Surgical excision of lung tissue.

Pneumonectomy: Surgical excision of entire lung.

Pneumoresection: Removal of a portion of a lung.

Lobectomy: Excision of a lobe.

Pleurectomy: Excision of a portion of the pleura.

Suture

Pneumonorrhaphy: Suture of the lung.

Endoscopy

Thoracoscopy: Exploratory examination of the chest by means of an endoscope.

Repair

Thoracoplasty: Plastic surgery of the thorax; operative repair of defects of the chest.

Thoracopneumoplasty: Plastic surgical operation of the chest and lung.

Surgical Collapse Therapy

Thoracocautery: Division by cautery of adhesions to complete the collapse of a lung in pneumothorax therapy.

CARDIOVASCULAR SYSTEM

For the life of the flesh is in the blood. LEVITICUS 17, 11

The cardiovascular system provides for the metabolic requirements of all the tissues of the body over a wide range of activity. The blood is a constant circulating fluid through the body (heart, arteries, veins and capillaries) conveying nutrition, food and oxygen, to the tissues and carrying away their waste products and carbon dioxide. Blood vessels are capable of changing their size in response to stimuli, so that circulation through any area may be increased or decreased in proportion to its activity, or to the activity of the body as a whole. Thus, the architecture and mechanisms of the cardiovascular system performs its role as the "obedient servant" of the body.

The heart, a hollow muscular organ, expels about 5 liters of blood a minute during rest and up to 35 liters of blood a minute during exercise. The heart is about the size of a closed fist, weighs about 10 ounces and is shaped like a blunt cone. As placed in the body, it has an oblique position, the right side is almost in front of the left, and about one-third of it is situated on the right and two-thirds on the left of the midline. The impulse of the heart against the chest wall is felt below the left nipple and about 3 inches (7.5 centimeters) to the left of the median line. The heart is enclosed in a double-walled membranous sac called the pericardium consisting of (1) an external fibrous portion and (2) an internal serous portion. This description is similar to that of visualizing a ball pushed into a slightly distended balloon: the inner layer adherent to the heart is called visceral pericardium; the layer forming the outer wall of the balloon is called the parietal pericardium. The inner surface of the cavities of the heart is lined by a serous membrane called the endocardium, which covers the valves, surrounds the chordae tendineae and is continuous with the lining membrane of the large blood vessels.

The main substance of the heart is cardiac muscle (myocardium). This tissue includes the muscle bundles of (1) the atria (auricles), (2) the ventricles, and (3) the conduction system.

The heart wall is formed by a mass of cardiac muscle fibers histologically unique in that it is a network of branching and anastomosing cylindrical fibers, striated but not voluntary in nature. The wall is lined by a delicate endocardium and invested by a layer of serous pericardium. The valves,

largely avascular except within their bases, are formed by a reduplication of the endocardium with a core of connective tissue. The dense fibrous rings and trigones of the orifices afford attachment to the cardiac fibers sweeping around the atria, on the one hand, and separately from the rest of the heart, there being no effective continuity between atrial and ventricular muscle except through a special atrioventricular bundle of modified cardiac cells.

The heart is divided into a right and left half by a muscular partition, the ventricular septum, extending from the base of the ventricles to the apex of the heart. These two sides have no communication with each other after birth. The right side contains venous blood and the left side arterial blood. Each half is divided into two cavities: the upper, atrium; the lower, ventricle. A spongework of muscle bars, the trabeculae carneae, project from the inner surface of the ventricles and are of three kinds, the first are attached along their entire length and form ridges, or columns; the second are situated at their extremities but are free in the middle; and the third are the superior and inferior papillary muscles which are continuous with the wall of each ventricle at its base. The aspices of these muscles gives rise to fibrous cords, the chordae tendineae, and are attached to the cusps of the atrioventricular valves.

VALVES OF HEART

The right atrioventricular valve, having three irregularly shaped flaps (cusps), is thus called tricuspid and separates the right atrium from the right ventricle. The valve is formed of fibrous tissue covered by endocardium. Continuous with one another at their bases, they form a ring-shaped membrane around the margin of the atrial openings. Their pointed ends project into the ventricle and are attached by the chordae tendineae to the papillary muscles, in the interior of the ventricles.

The pulmonic valve returns from the right ventricle to the main pulmonary artery. This valve has three cusps of equal size which form a perfect circle. The cusps are separated from the wall of the pulmonary artery.

The left atrioventricular valve consisting of two flaps or cusps is called the bicuspid or mitral valve and separates the left atrium from the left ventricle. It is attached in the same manner as the tricuspid valve. The valve permits the free flow of blood from the atria into the ventricles, but any flow forced backward is controlled by the flaps, an action of contracting and shortening of the papillary muscles to which the chordae tendineae are attached, and keep the chordae tendineae taut.

The aortic valve separates the left ventricle from the aorta. The aortic valve is very similar to the pulmonic valve in structure and appearance. The major difference is that two of the cusps give rise to the two coronary arteries.

ARTERIES

The arteries are distributed throughout the body in a systemic manner. Vessels leaving the heart are large but soon divide into branches, this division continuing until minute branches are distributed to all parts of the body (Plates 24-27). Branching and rebranching, the arteries become smaller and smaller, finally reaching the smallest arteries or arterioles, which run into the tiniest vessels, the capillaries.

DIVISION

Arteries divide in various ways:
1. Give off several branches in succession and still continue as a main trunk, e.g., the thoracic or abdominal portion of the aorta.
2. A short trunk may divide into several branches at the same time, e.g., the celiac artery.
3. An artery may divide into two branches of nearly equal size, e.g., the division of the aorta into the two common iliacs.
4. Distal ends of arteries unite at frequent intervals. Thus, they anastomose and permit free communication between the currents of the blood, prevent effects of local interruption and promote equality of distribution and pressure. Anastomoses occur between the larger as well as the smaller arteries.

Arteries have much thicker and stronger walls, but veins have the larger lumen related to their slower blood flow having to transport to time the same volume leaving the arterial system. Both have three coats, the tunica intima or endothelial lining, the tunica media, predominantly elastic in larger arteries, gradually replaced by muscle in arteries of medium size and entirely muscular in the small arteries and arterioles, and the tunica adventia, or fibrous coat, merging with the connective tissue bed in which the vessels lie. This different structure meets a functional need. The elastic distention of the aorta yields to, yet contains, the full force of the heart and in its recoil maintains the forward flow; the amount of elastic tissue, is a measure of the pressure to which an artery is subjected. Such arteries play a more passive role but arteries with muscular walls are rich in sympathetic nerves and dilate and contract in their particular control of the steady stream in the peripheral circulation.

VEINS

Veins withstand no serious pressure and have thin, mainly fibrous walls with little muscular and elastic tissue (Plates 28 and 29). (Nutrition is carried to the thicker walls of larger vessels by tiny arteries, vasa vasorum.)

The veins are distributed in two sets, superficial and deep veins. Three veins return the blood of the systemic circulation to the heart, namely, the coronary sinuses, the superior vena cava and the inferior vena cava.

The unique feature of the portal system is that the blood is detoured through the liver instead of being returned directly to the inferior vena cava.

PULMONARY CIRCULATION

Pulmonary circulation conveys the blood from the right ventricle of the heart to the lungs and back to the heart.

The pulmonary artery arises from the infundibulum of the right ventricle located in front of the aorta, both enclosed in a common tube of serous pericardium. At first, clasped on either side by the auricles and coronary arteries, it runs for 2 inches (5 cm) upwards and to the left in front of the left atrium, still within the fibrous pericardium, and then, under the aortic arch, divides into the right and left pulmonary arteries. The right pulmonary artery, passing in front of the esophagus and right bronchus, disappears behind the ascending aorta, the superior vena cava and the upper right pulmonary vein, and enters the root of the right lung to divide into an upper branch to the upper lobe and a lower branch to the middle and lower lobes.

The left pulmonary artery, smaller and, of course, shorter than the right, connected to the arch above by the ligamentum arteriosum, courses in front of the descending aorta, the left bronchus and the left vagus nerve to divide, in the root of the left lung, into branches to the upper and lower lobes. The terminal branches corresponding to the distribution of the bronchi.

The purpose of the pulmonary circulation is to carry blood which has circulated through the body and is returning to the heart loaded with tissue waste products and carbon dioxide, to the alveolar of the lungs. Here, the red cells are recharged with oxygen and carbon dioxide reduced to the standard amount.

The right atrium occupies the right border of the heart, crossed behind by the lower right pulmonary vein, and in part, lying in front of the left atrium.

The right ventricle, its wall only one-third as thick as that of the left ventricle, appears almost plastered to the side of the latter. The difference in thickness is accounted for by the greater amount of work the ventricles have to do as compared with the atria.

MOVEMENT OF BLOOD THROUGH RIGHT HEART AND LUNGS*

Superior, inferior venae cavae, coronary sinus—blood enters

↓

During diastole of the atria, via the superior and the inferior venae cavae, coronary sinus, and other small vessels, blood enters and fills the right atrium and ventricle, which for the time may be thought of as a single chamber with the tricuspid valve open.

Right atrium

↓

The atrium contracts (atrial systole) and forces the blood over the open valve into the ventricle, which has been passively filled and now becomes well distended by the extra supply.

Tricuspid valve

↓

After a brief pause (0.1 sec.) the ventricle contracts, and the blood gets behind the tricuspid valve and closes the valve.

Right ventricle

↓

Semilunar valve

↓

Pressure rises within the ventricle until it exceeds the pressure in the pulmonary artery and the pulmonary semilunar valve opens and blood moves on into the pulmonary artery.

Pulmonary artery Divides into two branches

↓

The pulmonary artery divides into the right and left branches and takes blood into the lungs.

Lungs

↓

Here blood passes through innumerable capillaries that surround the alveolae of the lungs. Blood gives up carbon dioxide and the red cells are recharged with oxygen.

Capillaries unite to form veins

↓

The venules unite to form larger veins until finally two pulmonary veins from each lung are formed.

Pulmonary veins

↓

These return the oxygenated blood to the heart and complete the pulmonary circulation.

Left atrium

*From Kimber, D. C., and Gray, C. E.: *Textbook of Anatomy and Physiology*, revised by C. E. Stackpole and L. C. Leavell, ed. 13. MacMillan Company, NewYork, 1957.

SYSTEMIC CIRCULATION

More extensive circulation from the left ventricle to all parts of the body and its return to the right atrium is called systemic circulation.

The purpose of systemic circulation is to carry oxygen and nutritional material to the tissues and absorb waste products from the tissues.

The left atrium is a flattened pouch, its upper left hand corner prolonged as an auricle around the side of the pulmonary trunk. It is intimately related to the esophagus, since it occupies most of the base of the heart.

Contraction of the left atrium sends the blood into the left distributing chamber of the heart, the left ventricle. It pumps the blood into the largest artery, the aorta large branches from which run to the head, the limbs and the viscera (internal organs, the abdominal organs).

The left ventricle is a thick-walled cone, its apex the apex of the heart, its base formed by the atrioventricular and aortic orifices.

After leaving the left ventricle, the blood flows in different courses, some portions entering the coronary arteries, some go to the head, some to the extremities and to the various internal organs. The longest journey the blood travels is from the left heart to the toes and back to the right heart, then to the lungs and to the left heart.

MOVEMENT OF BLOOD THROUGH LEFT HEART AND SOMATIC CAPILLARIES*

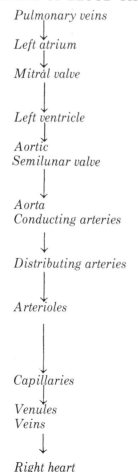

Pulmonary veins
↓
Left atrium
↓
Mitral valve

↓

Left ventricle
↓
Aortic
Semilunar valve

↓

Aorta
Conducting arteries

↓

Distributing arteries

↓

Arterioles

↓

Capillaries
↓
Venules
Veins

↓

Right heart

During diastole of the atria, oxygenated blood from the pulmonary veins enters the left atrium and fills it. The left ventricle relaxes and the pressure within it falls, the mitral valve opens and blood enters the ventricle and fills it. Systole of the atrium begins and ventricular filling is completed.

Blood gets behind the cusps of the mitral valve and closes them. Ventricular systole is initiated. Intraventricular pressure rises, and when it exceeds the pressure in the aorta the aortic semilunar valve opens and blood moves on into the aorta under high pressure.

Blood moves on into the conducting or elastic arteries (innominate, subclavian, common carotids, internal iliac, femoral).

Blood is forced onward by the recoil of these stretched elastic arteries into the distributing (muscular arteries) such as the axillary, radial, popliteal and tibial, and finally into the arterioles, where blood is moving in a steady stream, and then on into the capillaries, where the main work of the vascular bed is accomplished.

The capillaries unite to form venules and these in turn unite to form veins, then larger veins, until blood finally reaches the right atrium and the circuit begins again. This is known as systemic circulation.

*From Kimber, D. C., and Gray, C. E.: *Textbook of Anatomy and Physiology*, revised by C. E. Stackpole and L. C. Leavell, ed. 13. MacMillan Company, New York, 1957.

Systemic circulation then includes:

1. Coronary circulation

The left coronary artery supplies the left atrium and left ventricle, and may supply either the anterior half or the entire intraventriculary septum; the right coronary artery supplies the right atrium and the right ventricle adjoining the septum.

2. Circulation in upper extremity

The blood on its way to the arm, leaves the left ventricle of the heart through the ascending portion of the aorta and is returned to the right atrium by the superior vena cava.

3. Circulation in lower extremity

The blood that passes to the lower extremity leaves the left ventricle of the heart through the aorta and is returned to the right atrium by the inferior vena cava.

4. Circulation in organs of digestive system

Blood is supplied by the celiac, superior mesenteric and inferior mesenteric arteries.

5. Portal circulation

Circulation away from the heart and back again ordinarily involves only one set of capillaries. An exception is to be found in the vessels of the abdominal organs. Blood supplied to the spleen, pancreas, stomach and intestines by systemic arteries is collected into a large vein, the portal vein, which enters the liver and divides and spreads out into branches within it. Thus, as the blood courses through the capillary-like sinusoids, it exchanges nutrient materials with the liver cells, and is then collected into the hepatic veins which empty into the large systemic vena cava inferior just before it opens into the right atrium. This is portal circulation.

6. Carotid system

Principal arteries of blood supply to the head and neck are the two common carotids, each dividing into two branches: (1) the external carotid, which supplies the exterior of the head, the face and the greater part of the neck; (2) the internal carotid, which supplies to a great extent the parts within the cranial and orbital cavities.

Veins of the neck, which return the blood from the head and face are the external jugular, anterior jugular, posterior external jugular, internal jugular and the vertebral vein. Veins of the brain possess no valves, and because they have no muscular tissue their walls are extremely thin. These veins pierce the arachnoid membrane and inner or meningeal layer of the dura mater and open into the cranial venous sinuses. They are divided into two sets, the cerebral and cerebellar.

7. Renal circulation

Provision is made to remove impurities from the blood and also excessive amounts of water and of other nominal constituents by circulating the blood, via the renal arteries, amid a remarkable formation of secreting tubules in the kidneys. The kidneys play the role of filters and from here the blood returns via the renal veins to the systemic circulation. This circuit is known as the renal circulation.

8. Fetal circulation

Fetal circulation involves an arrangement by which an exchange of materials is effected between the blood of the embryo and that of the mother (Plate 30). The oxygenated blood from the placenta is carried to the embryo by the umbilical vein; the blood from the embryo is returned to the placenta by umbilical arteries. Nearly all the blood of the umbilical vein traverses the liver before entering the inferior vena cava, which accounts for the large size of the liver, particularly at an early period of fetal life. Fetal circulation is so perfectly adapted for the requirements of the fetus that only a few modifications are necessary for the adult circulation. Almost immediately when a child is born, the umbilical arteries close down, followed quickly by contraction of the umbilical vein and ductus venosus.

CONDUCTION SYSTEM

The conduction system initiates and superimposes a rhythm with a rapid rate which it transmits to all parts of the heart and one which can be regulated by the nervous system. Cardiac muscle which is capable of independent rhythmic action is normally coordinated by a special conduction system consisting of the sinoatrial node, which initiates and sends each atrial contraction wave to the atrioventricular node and bundle, which in turn receives and transmits the wave to the ventricles, the fine branches of the bundle, the terminal subendocardial network, which send the impulse from the apex over the ventricles. The dense network of very fine nerve fibers is an important part of the conducting system.

The autonomic nervous system innervating the heart is distributed mainly to the vessels and conduction system, stabilizing the cardiac contractions and adjusting them to the needs of the body, thus, the sympathetic accelerating, and the vagus braking. If the bundle becomes functionally blocked, the ventricles continue to beat but slower than and out of step with the atria.

CARDIAC CYCLE

The cardiac cycle is of two phases: (1) a period of contraction known as systole; (2) a period of dilation called the diastole. In man the average heart rate at rest is 70 to 72 beats per minute. The alternating dilation and contraction of an artery constitutes the pulse.

BLOOD PRESSURE

Blood pressure is the pressure the blood exerts against the walls of the vessels in which it is contained, including herein venous, arterial, and capillary pressure. However, it is most frequently applied to pressure existing in the large arteries, usually the left brachial artery just above the left elbow. The difference in arterial and venous pressure is best described by observing that a vein is easily flattened with a finger, an artery offers stronger resistance.

Systolic pressure is when blood pressure is highest in the arteries during the period of ventricular systole; diastolic pressure is the lowest pressure cardiac diastole causes in the brachial artery.

HEART ACTION

Blood pressure, emotional excitement or intense interest affect the frequency and strength of the heart beat as do reflex influences of an unconscious nature such as blood temperature; characteristics of heart muscle such as tone, irritability, contractility and conductivity; physical characteristics such as size, sex, age, posture and muscular exercise; changes in the condition of blood vessels and certain internal secretions.

BLOOD

Blood is the fluid medium which circulates through the arteries and veins transporting: (1) oxygen from the lungs to the tissues; (2) nutritive material absorbed from the intestine to the tissues; (3) products formed in one tissue to other tissues for use, e.g., hormones and internal secretions; and (4) waste products of metabolism to the organs of excretion—the lungs, kidneys, intestine and skin.

The blood functions to: (1) maintain body temperature at a normal level; (2) maintain a normal acid-base balance of the tissues; and (3) maintain a fluid balance between blood and tissues.

In an adult, blood volume constitutes about 1/12 or 1/13 of the body weight and plasma volume about 1/20 to 1/25 of body weight. Thus an individual weighing 154 lb. would contain about 6 quarts of blood.

COMPOSITION OF BLOOD

Blood consists of cells, or corpuscles, in an intercellular liquid called plasma;

Blood	Cells	Erythrocytes, or red cells
		White cells Lymphocytes
		Monocytes
		Granulocytes
		Platelets or thrombocytes
	Plasma	

The average number of formed elements in one cubic millimeter of blood are:

Erythrocytes	4,500,000 to 5,500,000
Leukocytes	6,000 to 10,000
Platelets	200,000 to 800,000

The differential count of white blood cells have the following averages:

Polymorphonuclear neutrophils	50 to 75%
Polymorphonuclear eosinophils	2 to 4%
Polymorphonuclear basophils	0.5%
Lymphocytes	20 to 40%
Monocytes	3 to 8%

Blood contains:

Water	78%		
Solids	22%	Proteins	18.5%
		Glucose	0.1
		Lipids (Fats)	1.4
		Salts (inorganic)	1.5
		Waste products	0.5%

CONSTITUENTS IN BLOOD*

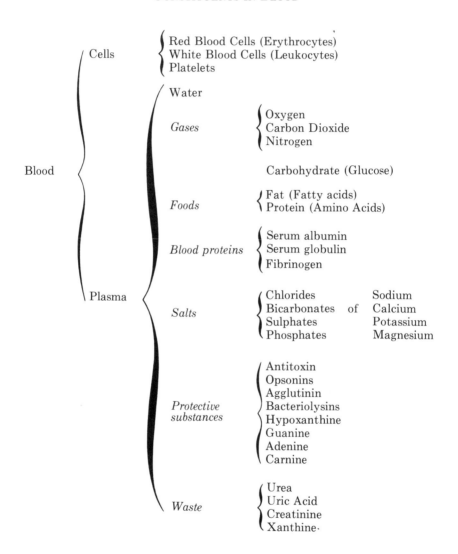

Blood
- Cells
  - Red Blood Cells (Erythrocytes)
  - White Blood Cells (Leukocytes)
  - Platelets
- Plasma
  - Water
  - *Gases*
    - Oxygen
    - Carbon Dioxide
    - Nitrogen
  - *Foods*
    - Carbohydrate (Glucose)
    - Fat (Fatty acids)
    - Protein (Amino Acids)
  - *Blood proteins*
    - Serum albumin
    - Serum globulin
    - Fibrinogen
  - *Salts*
    - Chlorides
    - Bicarbonates   of
    - Sulphates
    - Phosphates
    - Sodium
    - Calcium
    - Potassium
    - Magnesium
  - *Protective substances*
    - Antitoxin
    - Opsonins
    - Agglutinin
    - Bacteriolysins
    - Hypoxanthine
    - Guanine
    - Adenine
    - Carnine
  - *Waste*
    - Urea
    - Uric Acid
    - Creatinine
    - Xanthine.

*From Taber's Cyclopedic Medical Dictionary, ed. 10. F. A. Davis Company, Philadelphia, 1964.

SURGICAL PROCEDURES— CARDIOVASCULAR SYSTEM

Heart and Pericardium

Incision

Cardiotomy: Incision of the heart.

Pericardiostomy: Formation of an opening into the pericardium for drainage.

Pericardiotomy: Incision of a membranous sac around the heart.

Pericardiocentesis: Puncture of the pericardial space for aspiration.

Valvulotomy or commissurotomy: Process of cutting through a valve or commissure.

Excision

Pericardiectomy: Excision of part or all of the pericardium.

Cardiovalvulotomy: The excision of part of a valve, especially for mitral valve.

Destruction

Cardiolysis: Surgical procedure to free pericardial adhesions from surrounding tissues, involving resection of the ribs and sternum.

Pericardiolysis: Separation of adhesions between the visceral and parietal pericardium.

Suture

Cardiorrhaphy: Suturing of the heart muscle.

Pericardiorrhaphy: Suturing of a pericardial wound or injury.

Arteries and Veins

Incision

Arteriotomy: Surgical division or opening of an artery.

Phlebotomy: The opening of a vein, venesection.

Excision

Phlebectomy: Excision of a vein, or a part of a vein.

Introduction

Arteriography: Roentgenography of arteries after injection of radiopaque material into the bloodstream.

Venography: Roentgenograph of veins.

Blood transfusion: Indirect method, replacement type, RH factor; direct method.

Intravenous: For introduction of medication.

Repair

Repair of aortic arch anomalies.

Anastomosis: An operative procedure to unite two hollow or tubular structures, e.g., blood vessels.

Aortic anastomosis: (1) *Pott's anastomosis*—Pulmonary aortic anastomosis. This procedure is a direct side-to-side anastomosis between the aorta and the pulmonary artery as a palliative procedure in Fallot's tetralogy. (2) *Blalock-Taussig pulmonary subclavian anastomosis*—In congenital malformations of the heart, e.g., stenosis at the pulmonary orifice and a septal defect with cyanosis, wherein an abnormally small volume of blood passes through the pulmonary circuit. Thus, blood from the systemic circulation is directed to the lungs by anastomosing the innominate, right or left subclavian or a carotid artery to the pulmonary artery.

Venous Anastomosis: Portacaval anastomosis; splenorenal anastomosis; plastic operation for repair of arteriovenous aneurysm.

Suture

Arteriorrhaphy: Suture of wound or injury of an artery.

Phleborrhaphy: Suture of wound or injury of a vein.

Ligation: The application of a ligature (for tying a vessel).

LYMPHATIC SYSTEM

Its biting lymph may not be touch'd of man / Or God, unless the fates have so ordain'd. ROBERT BRIDGES, EROS & PSYCHE, DEC. XXIX

The lymphatic system consists of lymphatic capillaries, the lymphatic vessels and the lymph nodes or glands.

The system begins in meshes of connective tissues as closed capillaries, thin-walled tubes, composed of a single layer of endothelial cells, which anastomose to form networks, and contains lymph, a colorless fluid, much like blood plasma but rich in cells, particularly lymphocytes, which go to the regional lymph nodes. These capillaries form the first collecting trunks or afferent vessels. Lymph capillaries join to make lymphatic vessels which possess numerous paired valves, giving them a closely beaded appearance. The lymph flows from the lymphatic capillaries in all parts of the body into the lymphatic vessels, which are like the veins in structure. In their course, the larger lymphatic vessels drain into lymph nodes or glands and finally come together to form two large trunks, the right lymphatic duct and the thoracic duct, which enter the great veins at the root of the neck. The lymph nodes aggregate in the groin, axilla and neck (Plates 31 and 32).

The right lymphatic duct is the smaller of the two. It carries the lymph from the right arm, right side of thorax and right side of the head and neck, and empties into the right brachiocephalic vein, where it arises from the union of the right internal jugular and subclavian vein.

The thoracic duct carries the lymph from all the remaining parts of the body and empties it into the left brachiocephalic vein. The thoracic duct begins on the posterior abdominal wall at the lower border of the second lumbar vertebra in a pouch-like dilation called the cisterna chyle, continuing upward along the bodies of the vertebrae to its termination.

MOVEMENT OF LYMPH

The lymph flows from the tissues toward the lymphatic ducts. The flow is maintained chiefly by the difference in pressure of the two ends of the system. The low pressure end is at the beginning of the large ducts into the brachiocephalic veins at the other end. In the region of the lymphatic capillaries the pressure is high. Accessory factors aiding the flow of lymph are breathing movements and muscular contractions. Respiratory movements aspirate lymph into the veins in the upper chest region. The lymph vessels are alternately compressed and released by the contraction and relaxation of skeletal muscle.

The lymph nodes or glands are oval or bean-shaped bodies located at rather frequent intervals along the course of a lymph vessel. The lymph nodes are usually distributed in groups. *In the Head and Neck:* (1) submaxillary nodes, just below the angle of the mandible; (2) preauricular nodes, just in front of the ear; (3) postauricular, behind the ear in the region of the mastoid process; (4) the superficial cervical nodes, at the side of the neck, over the sternocleidomastoid muscle; (5) the deep cervical nodes, deep in the neck along the carotid artery and internal jugular vein.

The main group of the upper extremity is in the axilla (armpit), and receives lymph from the arm, anterior and lateral walls of the chest, mammary gland and scapular region.

The most important glands of the lower extremity are the inguinal nodes, which lie in the groin. They receive the lymph from the leg and the external genitalia.

Important groups in the thoraco-abdominal cavity are tracheobronchial, mediastinal, gastric, mesenteric and numerous glands along the main arterial trunks.

The spleen is the largest mass of lymphatic tissue in the body. An ovoid soft, friable, purple, contractile organ about $4^1/_2$ inches long (12 cm), it is located on the left side of the abdominal cavity. Its lateral surface is convex and lies molded against the dome of the diaphragm. It varies in size in different persons, and even in the same person under different conditions. It increases during digestion and is smaller with starvation. A normal weight being about 6 ounces. The medial surface is in contact with the stomach, the pancreas and the left kidney. The spleen is placed in the course of the blood circulation through the splenic artery and in many respects it acts as a filter and a reservoir for the blood.

The spleen manufactures all types of blood cells during fetal life, and for a short time after birth. In adult life this function is restricted to the formation of lymphocytes and monocytes.

Principal function of the spleen is the

production of antibodies, as well as the destruction of red blood corpuscles, and preparation of new hemoglobin from the iron.

SURGICAL PROCEDURES— LYMPHATIC SYSTEM

Spleen
Excision
Splenectomy: Surgical removal of the spleen.

Lymph Nodes and Lymphatic Channels
Incision
Drainage of lymph node abscess (lymphadenitis).
Excision
Biopsy of lymph nodes, e.g., anterior scalene.
Excision of lymph node.
Radical lymphadenectomy: Radical resection of lymph nodes in upper neck, axilla, cervical, unilateral or bilateral (suprahyoid or complete), groin.

Mediastinum
Incision
Mediastinotomy: Incision into the mediastinum.
Excision
Excision of mediastinal cyst.
Excision of mediastinal tumor.
Repair thoracic duct (suture).
Plastic anastomosis of the thoracic duct.

GENITOURINARY SYSTEM

Sirrah . . . what says the doctor to my water? FALSTAFF, HENRY IV, PART II, SHAKESPEARE

. . . and they shall be one flesh. GENESIS 2, 25

The urinary system consists of a pair of kidneys which secrete urine, a pair of ureters, or tubes that convey urine to the urinary bladder which temporarily stores the urine, and a urethra through which the urine is discharged from the body.

KIDNEYS

The kidneys are sensitive filters, with a remarkable arrangement of blood vessels and tubules (small canals) adjusting the water balance of the body and eliminating impurities and excess in the urine. They are placed at the back of the abdominal cavity, one on each side of the spinal column and behind the peritoneum. This position corresponds to the space between the upper border of the twelfth thoracic vertebra and the third lumbar vertebra. The right kidney is a little lower than the left due to the large space occupied by the liver.

The kidneys are large brown bodies about 4 inches long, 2 inches wide and 1 inch thick, with the medial or concave border directed toward the medial line of the body. On this border is a deep excavation in the substance of the organ called the renal sinus, the opening of which is the hilus of the kidney (which gives the kidney its bean-like shape) and serves as a passageway for the ureter and for the blood vessels, lymph vessels and nerves going to and from the kidney. The convex border of the kidney is on the lateral side. The thin, smooth covering of the kidney is called the renal capsule. Outside this capsule is connective and fatty tissue known as the adipose capsule. A fibrous layer encloses the kidney and perirenal fat, Gerota's capsule, and helps maintain the kidney in its normal position.

In man the entire blood volume (5 1/2 liters) passes through the kidneys 15 times an hour, so that renal blood flow is 75 liters an hour. The blood is filtered by Malphigian bodies or glomeruli, surrounded by Bowman's capsule which collects the filtrate into *renal tubules*. These glomeruli lie in the *renal cortex*. The tubules, ascending and descending loops (of Henle) concentrate the urine and form the pyramids of the medulla, and the apex of each pyramid, pierced by tubular openings, lies in a calyx or cup of the collecting system. This functional unit, glomerulus and tubule is called a nephron. Groups of calyces drain through infundibula into the renal pelvis and so to the ureter.

The ureters are tubes about 10 inches long (27 cm), which carry the urine to the bladder. Each ureter is composed of three layers, an inner or mucous coat covered with transitional, stratified epithelieum, a middle coat of smooth muscle with inner circular and outer longitudinal layers, and an outer fibrous coat. Peristaltic contractions of the ureters transport urine to the bladder.

URINARY BLADDER

The urinary bladder is a hollow, dilatable muscular sac lying in the pelvis behind the symphysis pubis, in front of the rectum above the prostate gland in the male, and in front of the vagina and uterus in the female. It serves as a reservoir in which urine is retained until it is eliminated from the body.

Normally the bladder is emptied when it contains about a half a pint, although it can contain 20 ounces without too much discomfort.

On the floor of the bladder lies a triangle of muscle, the trigone, with a ureter entering at each posterior corner and the internal urethra orifice at the apex in front.

URETHRA

In the female the urethra is a simple tube 1 1/2 inches long (3.5 cm) passing down behind the symphysis, through the urogenital diaphragm and emptying between the labia minora, in front of the vagina and below the clitoris; as it passes through the urogenital diaphragm, it is surrounded by striated muscle, the voluntary sphincter of the membranous urethra. The wall of the urethra has an inner mucous membrane layer, a thin submucous coat and a thick muscular layer.

The male urethra is 7 inches long (20 cm), and is composed of three portions: prostatic, membranous, and penile or cavernous. The prostatic urethra extends from the bladder neck to the pelvic floor. It is 1 inch long and is surrounded by the pros-

tate gland. The membranous urethra is that portion which pierces the muscular pelvic floor and is 1/2 inch long. The penile urethra, in the groove ventral to the corpora cavernosa penis, is proximally fixed by the suspensory ligament of the penis, and distally pendulous. This gives the male urethra the S-shaped curve which differs from the short, straight course of the female urethra, making instrumentation more difficult.

URINE
"Description"

Volume:	Average—1500 cc /24 hours.
Color:	Pale yellow due to pigment, urobilin.
pH:	(or H ion concentration) 4.5 (acid) to 8 (alkaline) depending upon diet.
S.G.:	(Specific gravity) 1.004 to 1.030 depending on fluid load or abnormal constituents, e.g., sugar. Night urine is highly concentrated.
Solids:	*Inorganic Compounds:* urea, sodium chloride, the sulfates, phosphates of sodium, potassium, magnesium, and calcium. *Organic Compounds:* urea, uric acid, creatinine, and ammonium salts.

Micturition

Urine is secreted continuously by the kidneys. It is carried to the bladder by the ureters and at intervals is expelled through the urethra. The act by which the urine is expelled is called micturition. The desire to urinate is due to sensory stimulation in the bladder itself, caused by pressure of urine or reflex stimulation. The act is essentially a reflex through the central nervous system.

There are three types of micturition:

1. Involuntary or incontinence may occur as the result of lack of consciousness, or as a result of spinal injury involving the nerve centers which send nerves of control to the bladder. In young infants, incontinence of urine is normal. Retention of urine: (1) may occur as the result of an obstruction in the urethra or neck of the bladder; (2) nervous contraction of the urethra; or

(3) by the dulling of senses.

2. Suppression of urine, or anuria, is the failure of the kidneys to secrete urine.

3. Frequency of urine, or oliguria, is the diminished secretion of urine, and frequency of urination.

Formation of Urine

The first step in the formation of urine occurs in the glomeruli. An ultrafiltrate of plasma, composed of water and nonprotein solutes, passes through the glomerular membranes into Bowman's Capsules and thence into the proximal tubules. The pressure for filtration is supplied by the work of the heart.

The urinary system is shown in Plate 33.

GENITAL SYSTEM

MALE GENITAL ORGANS

The male genital system includes the testes which produce both the male hormones and the male germ cells, called spermatozoa, with their ducts for transporting the spermatozoa, the epididymis and ductus deferens (vas deferens), the prostate gland, the bulbourethral glands, the penis, the scrotum and the urethra.

The testes are two ovoid bodies, right and left, lying in the scrotum which produce the male cells or spermatozoa. The spermatozoa escape successfully through the epididymis, vas deferens, ejaculatory duct and the urethra to the meatus of the penis. The penis with the scrotum and its contents are termed the external genitalia.

FEMALE GENITAL ORGANS

The female genital system consists of two ovaries, which produce the female germ cells or ova and in which sex cells develop; two uterine tubes, through which the sex cells pass; the vagina, a canal that connects the uterus or womb, a thick walled, muscular, pear-shaped organ, about 3 inches long between the bladder and rectum, comprising an upper part, the cervix, which projects into the anterior wall of the vagina, the uterus being almost at right angles to that of the vagina, to the exterior; and the external genitalia composed of the mons pubis, labia majora, which border the pudendal cleft, the labia minora, the clitoris, bulb of the vestibule and the vestibular glands. The mammary glands are accessory organs of the female reproductive system. The male and female genital systems are shown in Plate 33.

The human organism begins life as a single-celled embryo, derived from the fusion of pre-existing parental cells, the ovum and the spermatozoon. This one-celled embryo undergoes repeated mitotic cell division, forming the multicellular organism.

The life cycle of man is divided into two periods, prenatal life and postnatal life.

Prenatal life: (1) period of ovum—first 2 weeks of development; (2) embryonic period—from the beginning of the 3rd week to the end of the second month; (3) fetal period—from the beginning of the 3rd month to the time of birth.

Postnatal life: (1) neonatal period—from birth to the end of the second week; (2) infancy—from the second week to the end of the first year; (3) childhood—from the end of infancy to puberty, which comes at about the twelfth to the sixteenth year. Puberty is indicated in the male by production of functional spermatozoa; in the female by the onset of ovulation and menstruation. (4) adolescence—extending from puberty into the early or middle twenties; (5) maturity—early and middle maturity lasting from adolescence to the end of the reproductive period, followed by late maturity.

SURGICAL PROCEDURES— URINARY SYSTEM

Kidney

Incision

Drainage of perirenal abscess.

Nephrotomy: Incision (not exploratory) of the kidney.

Nephrostomy: Formation of an artificial fistula into the renal pelvis.

Nephrolithotomy: Surgical renal incision for removal of calculus.

Division or transection of aberrant renal vessels.

Pyelotomy: Surgical incision into the renal pelvis.

Pyelostomy: Surgical creation of an opening into the renal pelvis.

Pyelolithotomy: Surgical removal of calculus from the pelvis of a kidney through an incision.

Excision

Renal biopsy.

Nephrectomy: Removal of a kidney, may include excision of a ureter. Total or partial ureterectomy.

Excision of cyst of kidney.

Aspiration of a renal cyst.

Renal sympathectomy: Excision of renal sympathetic nerve.

Introduction

Perirenal insufflation, unilateral or bilateral.

Repair

Nephrolysis: A surgical detachment of an inflamed kidney from adhesions.

Pyeloplasty: Plastic operation on renal pelvis, with or without plastic operation on ureter.

Pyelocystostomosis: Formation of a surgical communication between the kidney and the bladder.

Nephropexy: Surgical attachment of a floating kidney.

Suture

Repair of ruptured kidney.

Nephrorrhaphy: Suture of a floating kidney to the posterior wall of the abdomen.

Closure of a renal fistula.

Ureter

Incision

Ureterotomy: Surgical incision of the ureter.

Ureterolithotomy: Surgical incision for removal of a calculus from a ureter.

Excision

Ureteronephrectomy: Complete or partial excision of a ureter.

Ureteronephrectomy: Surgical removal of a kidney and its ureter.

Ureteroenterostomy: Surgical formation of a passage between a ureter and the intestine, unilateral or bilateral.

Repair

Ureteroplasty: Plastic surgery of the ureter.

Ureteropyelostomy: Excision of a portion of the ureter with attachment the renal pelvis.

Ureterocystostomy: Artificial formation of an opening from the ureter into the bladder; unilateral or bilateral.

Ureteroproctostomy: Surgical formation of a passage from the ureter to the anus.

Ureterostomy: Formation of a permanent fistula for drainage of a ureter.

Ureterosigmoidostomy: Surgical implantation of ureter into the sigmoid colon.

Suture

Ureterorrhaphy: Suture or suspension of the ureter.

Bladder

Incision

Cystectasy: Surgical extraction of a calculus from the bladder, and the dilation of the bladder.

Puncture aspiration of bladder by needle.

Cystostomy: Surgical incision into the bladder.

Puncture aspiration.

Cystotomy: Incision of bladder.

Cystolithectomy: Surgical excision of a calculus by cutting into the bladder.

Drainage of perivesical or perivesical space abscess.

Cystotrachelotomy: Surgical incision into neck of the bladder.

Excision

Transurethral electroresection of vesical neck, female.

Excision of bladder diverticulum.

Excision of bladder tumor.

Transurethral resection of bladder tumors.

Repair

Cystoplasty: Plastic surgery upon the bladder.

Cystorectostomy: Formation of a surgical communication between the bladder and rectum.

Endoscopy

Cystoscopy: Diagnostic; with or without biopsy, with or without urethral catheterization.

Cystoscopy with fulguration of minor lesion of the bladder.

Cystoscopy with fulguration of a bladder tumor.

Manipulation of uteric calculus.

Resection of fulguration of a ureterocele.

Destruction

Litholapaxy: The operation of crushing a stone in the bladder, followed by immediate removal of fragments through a catheter, or cystoscope.

Suture

Repair of ruptured bladder.

Cystorrhaphy: Suture of bladder.

Closure of vesicovaginal, vesicouterine, or vesicorectal fistula.

Incision

Urethrotomy: Incision of a urethra, e. g. stricture.

Urethrostomy: Surgical formation of a permanent fistulous opening into the urethra.

Meatotomy: Cutting of the meatus.

Drainage of periurethral abscess.

Drainage of perineal urinary extravasation.

Excision

Urethrectomy: Surgical excision of the urethra or parts of it.

Excision of urethral caruncle or fulguration.

Excision of carcinoma of urethra.

Excision of diverticulum of urethra.

Excision of fulguration urethral polyps

Repair

Urethroplasty: Plastic operation repair of urethra.

Suture

Urethraorrhaphy: Suture of urethra.

Closure of urethrostomy or fistula of urethra.

Closure of urethrovaginal fistula.

MALE GENITAL SYSTEM

Penis

Incision

Dorsal or lateral slit of prepuce.

Excision

Biopsy of penis.

Amputation of penis, partial, complete, or radical.

Local excision of lesion of penis.

Circumcision: Removal of prepuce.

Excision (or fulguration) of *tissue.*

Repair

Plastic operation on penis for hypospadias, a congenital opening of urethra on dorsum of penis.

Urethroplasty: Plastic surgical repair of urethra.

Plastic operation on penis for injury, for epispadias or for urinary extravasation.

Testis

Incision

Orchidotomy: Surgical incision into testes.

Excision

Biopsy

Orchidectomy: Surgical excision of a testicle.

Repair

Surgical reduction of torsion of testis.

Orchioplasty: Plastic repair of the testicle.

Orchidoplasty: Operative transfer of an undescended testicle to the scrotum.

Orchiopexy: Surgical transfer of an imperfect descended testicle into the scrotum and suturing it there.

Orchiorrhaphy: Suturing of undescended testicle in the scrotum.

Epididymis

Incision

Epididymotomy: Incision into epididymis.

Excision

Epididymectomy: Surgical excision of epididymis.

Repair

Epididymovasostomy: Formation of an anastomosis between epididymis and vas deferens.

Tunical Vaginalis

Incision

Puncture aspiration of hydrocele.

Hydrocelectomy: Excision of various lesions.

Scrotum

Incision

Drainage of scrotal abscess.

Removal of foreign body in scrotum.

Excision

Scrotectomy: Surgical excision of part of the scrotum.

Local excision of lesion of scrotum.

Scrotoplasty: Plastic operation on scrotum.

Vas Deferens

Incision

Vasopuncture: Puncture of the vas deferens.

Vasotomy: Surgical incision of the vas deferens.

Vasostomy: Surgical formation of an opening into the vas deferens.

Excision

Vasectomy: Surgical removal of all or part of the vas deferens.

Vasoepididymostomy: Surgical formation of a passage between the vas deferens and the epididymis.

Repair

Vasovasostomy, re-anastomosis.

Suture

Vasorrhaphy: Surgical suture of vas deferens.

Spermatic Cord

Excision

Spermectomy: Resection of a part of the spermatic cord and duct.

Varicocelectomy: Excision of varicocele.

Seminal Vesicles

Incision

Spermatocystotomy: Surgical incision into a seminal vesicle for drainage.

Vesiculotomy: Incision into a vessel, e.g. seminal vesicle.

Excision

Spermatocystectomy: Removal of the seminal vesicles

Vesiculectomy: Partial or complete excision of a seminal vesicle.

Vesiculotomy: Surgical division of a seminal vesicle.

Prostate

Incision

Prostatocystotomy: Surgical incision of the prostate and the bladder.

Prostatotomy: Incision into the prostate gland.

Prostatolithotomy: Removal of prostatic calculus.

Prostatomy: Incision into the prostate.

Prostate-needle biopsy.

Excision

Prostatectomy: Surgical excision of prostate.

Prostatomyomectomy: Surgical excision of a prostatic myoma.

Prostatovesiculectomy: Surgical removal of the prostate gland and seminal vesicles.

FEMALE GENITAL SYSTEM

Vulva

Incision

Episiotomy: Incision of peritoneum at end of second stage of labor so as to avoid laceration of the perineum.

Incision and drainage of abscess of vulva.

Incision and drainage of Bartholin's gland, for abscess.

Hymenotomy: Incision of the hymen.

Clitoridotomy: Incision of the clitoris.

Excision

Clitoridectomy: Surgical excision of clitoris.

Biopsy of vulva.

Vulvectomy: Surgical excision of vulva.

Hymenectomy: Surgical removal of hymen.

Excision of fulguration of Skene's glands which lie just inside of and on the posterior floor of the urethra.

Repair

Episioplasty: Plastic surgery repair on the vulva.

Hymenorrhaphy: Plastic surgery operation on the hymen.

Suture

Episiorrhaphy: Surgical suturing of a lacerated perineum.

Episioperineorrhaphy: Surgical suturing of the vulva and for support of a prolapse of the uterus.

Vagina

Incision

Colpoceliotomy: Surgical incision into abdomen through the vagina.

Colpocystotomy: Surgical incision into bladder through the vagina.

Colpoureterotomy: Incision into ureter through the vagina.

Colpohysterectomy: Surgical removal of uterus through the vagina.

Excision

Biopsy of vagina.

Colpectomy: Surgical excision of part of the vagina.

Repair

Colpocystoplasty: Surgical treatment of vesico vaginal fistula.

Colpoplasty: Plastic surgery involving the vagina.

Colpoperineoplasty: Plastic operation on perineum and involving the vagina.

Suture

Colporrhaphy: (Elytrorrhaphy). Suture of a rupture of the vagina, by freshening and suturing the edges of the tear.

Colpoperineorrhaphy: Surgical repair by suture of perineal tears in vagina.

Oviduct (Fallopian tube or Uterine tube)

Incision

Salpingostomy: Surgical opening into a fallopian tube.

Salpingostomatomy: Surgical creation of an artificial opening in a fallopian tube.

Excision

Salpingectomy: Excision of an oviduct.

Salpingo-oophorectomy: Excision of an ovary and its fallopian tube.

Repair

Salpingosalpingostomy: Anastomosing one oviduct with its fellow on the other side; or re-anastomose a fallopian tube.

Suture

Salpingorraphy: Surgical suture of an oviduct.

Ovary

Incision

Ovariostomy: Surgical creation of an opening in an ovarian cyst or abscess, for drainage.

Ovariotomy: Incision into or removal of an ovary, or of an ovarian cyst.

Excision

Salpingo-ovariectomy: Surgical removal of an ovary and an oviduct.

Oophorectomy: Excision of an ovary.

Oophorohysterectomy: Surgical removal of uterus and ovaries.

Oothecectomy: Ablation of an ovary.

Ovariohysterectomy: Excision of the ovaries and uterus.

Ovariosalpingectomy: Excision of an ovary and an oviduct.

Oothecohysterectomy: Excision of the uterus and ovaries.

Suture

Oophoropeliopexy: Fixation of a prolapsed ovary by suturing it to the wall of the pelvis.

Oophoropexy: Fixation of a displaced ovary.

Oophorrhaphy: Suturing of a displaced ovary to the pelvic wall.

Uterus and Cervix Uteri

Incision

Hysterocervicotomy: Cesarean section.

Excision

Biopsy of cervix or endometrium.

Hysterectomy: Surgical removal of the uterus.

Hysteromyomectomy: Excision of a uterine myoma.

Hysteromyomotomy: Uterine incision for removal of a tumor.

Panhysterectomy: Total hysterectomy (corpus and cervix).

Hysterosalpingostomy: Anastomosis of the uterus with the distal portion of the fallopian tube, after excision of a mesial portion.

Cervicectomy: Surgical removal of the cervix uteri.

Local excision of lesion of cervix (cauterization or conization).

Hystero-oophorectomy: Surgical removal of the uterus and both ovaries.

Hysterosalpingo-oophorectomy: Surgical removal of uterus, oviducts and ovaries.

Dilatation and curettage.

Conization: Excision of a cone of tissue, e.g., mucosa of the cervix.

Repair

　Hysteropexy: Abdominal fixation of uterus.

Perineum

Incision

　Perineotomy: Incision of the perineum.

　Perineoplasty: Plastic surgical repair of the perineum.

Repair

　Perineorrhaphy: Plastic surgery of the perineum.

Maternity:
Fetus and Fetal Structures

Incision

　Cesarotomy: Classic cesarean section; Removal of the fetus by means of an incision into the uterus through the abdominal wall.

Excision

　Removal of extrauterine embryo (ectopic pregnancy) by laparotomy.

OBSTETRICAL PROCEDURES

Obstetric procedures.

Obstetrical delivery, including ante partum and post partum care.

Miscarriage or abortion before period of viability, including prenatal care, and including dilation and curettage.

Therapeutic abortion by dilatation and curettage of uterus.

Dilatation and curettage of uterus for postpartum bleeding.

Hystero-oophorectomy: Surgical removal of the uterus and one or both ovaries.

Hysterosalpingo-oophorectomy: Surgical removal of uterus, oviducts and ovaries.

DIGESTIVE SYSTEM

In the sweat of thy face shalt thou eat bread; til those return unto the ground, for out of it wast thou taken; for dust thou art. GENESIS 3, 19

The digestive system consists of the alimentary canal, a musculomembranous tube about 30 feet (9 meters) long extending from the mouth to the anus, and a number of related organs. Except for the first 12 inches down to the stomach, all of the digestive tract is in the abdominal cavity along with the important accessory organs, the liver and pancreas. The digestive tract is concerned with elaborating foods into forms suitable for absorption into the blood stream followed by storage and assimilation by the tissues.

The digestive system as explained in this chapter is outlined under the following headings:

1. Mouth, oral or buccal cavity, which contains the tongue, orifices of ducts of the salivary glands.
2. Salivary glands.
3. Teeth and muscles of mastication.
4. Pharynx.
5. Esophagus.
6. Stomach.
7. Small intestine; divided into three por-

tions, the duodenum, jejunum and ileum. The ileocecal valve is the passageway from the small to the large intestine.

8. Large intestine, which is divided into the cecum, ascending colon, transverse colon, descending colon, sigmoid colon, rectum and anal canal. The first five of these subdivisions are often spoken of jointly as the "colon." With the rectum, they compose the "colorectum."
9. Rectum.
10. Anal canal.
11. Accessory organs of digestion are the salivary glands, liver, gallbladder and pancreas.

Ingestion of food and water is one of the essential homeostatic (stabilizing) mechanisms for maintenance of the energy balance and the constancy of the internal environment of the body. Hunger, appetite and satiety, which regulate food intake, are actually functions of the central nervous system, more specifically of the hypothalamus.

Food is chewed in the mouth, then swallowed via the pharynx and esophagus through the neck and thorax into the abdomen, where the stomach digests a whole meal to a certain stage before its transmission to the small intestines for further digestion and absorption. The residue passes in a semifluid state through the ileocecal valve into the last part of the intestine, the large intestine, for absorption of water and retention of residue until excreted through the anus. The abdominal and thoracic viscera are shown in Plates 34 and 35.

MOUTH

The mouth, oral or buccal cavity is a cavity bound laterally in front by the cheeks and the lips, which form the anterior boundary and the glossopalatine arch the posterior limit, at which point it leads into the pharynx. The roof is formed by the palate, the floor by the tongue. It houses the teeth, which are embedded in the upper and lower jaws. The tongue is a muscular organ, and is the special organ of the sense of taste.

SALIVARY GLANDS

Salivary glands secrete saliva, a clear fluid which moistens food and also contains an enzyme which digests cooked starch. Numerous small mucous and serous glands, labial, buccal, palatine and lingual, constantly moisten the membrane of the mouth with a jelly-like lubricating mucous secretion diluted by a thin, watery serous fluid. The salivary glands are arranged in pairs, the parotid (on the cheeks in front of the ears), the submandibular (submaxillary, under the jaws) and the sublingual glands.

TEETH

Thirty-two permanent teeth are the organs of mastication. The four muscles of mastication are the masseter, temporal, external pterygoid, and internal pterygoid muscles, aided by certain accessory muscles of which the buccinator is the most important.

PHARYNX

The pharynx is a funnel-shaped cavity with fibromuscular walls attached to the base of the skull above and continuous with the esophagus below at the level of the cricoid cartilage opposite the sixth cervical vertebrae. It may be divided into three parts. The upper part, or nasopharynx, lies behind the nose and is an air passage only; the middle part or oropharynx lies behind the mouth, serving both the respiratory and digestive tracts as a common pathway; and the lower part or laryngopharynx lies behind the larynx and is a pathway for food passing into the esophagus.

ESOPHAGUS

The esophagus, or gullet, is a muscular tube approximately 10 inches (25 cm) long which conveys food from the pharynx to the stomach. It lies posterior to the trachea and the heart and just in front of the vertebrae. In the lower part of its course it sweeps in front of the aorta, passing through the diaphragm at the left of the median line to end in the stomach.

STOMACH

In the abdominal cavity, the esophagus ends in the stomach (gaster) a dilated portion of the alimentary canal lying in the left upper quadrant, hypochondriac and epigastric abdominal regions. The stomach serves as a temporary receptacle for food while digestion proceeds. The shape and position of the stomach are modified by changes within itself and in the surrounding organs. These modifications are determined by the amount of the stomach contents, the stage of digestion which has been reached, the degree of development and power of the muscular walls and the condition of the adjacent intestine.

The opening from the esophagus into the stomach is called the cardiac orifice, since it is just below the heart; and the exit from the stomach into the small intestine is called the pyloric orifice. The two borders of the stomach pass between these orifices. The right border or lesser curvature is short and somewhat concave; the left border or greater curvature is long and convex.

The stomach is composed of a central portion, the body, a balloon-like portion; the fundus, an upper portion, to the left and above; and a constricted lower portion to the right and below, the antrum.

The fundus and body secrete acid and

pepsin; the antrum secretes gastrin (see P. 87) a hormone which stimulates the fundus and body to secrete more acid and pepsin.

A notch on the lesser curvature, the incisura angularis, marks off the body from the antrum. The mucous membrane is smooth when the stomach is full, but is thrown into folds, called rugae, when empty.

SMALL INTESTINE

The small intestine, a coiled 20-foot (7-meter) tube occupying the central and lower abdomen, practically completes the digestion of the food and passes the semifluid contents through the ileocecal orifice in the right iliac fossa into the large intestine.

The small intestine is divided into three portions: the duodenum, the jejunum and the ileum. The duodenum is 10 inches (25 cm) long, is attached to the posterior abdominal wall and arranged in a horseshoe-shape to enclose the head of the pancreas. The bile and pancreatic ducts open into the duodenum about 4 inches (8 to 10 cm) from the pylorus. The jejunum is 7 1/2 feet (2.2 meters) long, and it continues from the duodenum, thence to the ileum, 10 to 14 feet (between 3 and 4 meters) long, which connects with the large intestine at the cecum. The jejunum and ileum are attached to the posterior abdominal wall by an extensive fold of peritoneum, the mesentery, which allows the freest motion, permitting each coil to accommodate itself to changes in form and position.

LARGE INTESTINE

The remaining portion of the alimentary canal is the large intestine, approximately 5 feet (1.5 meters) long, divided into the cecum, colon, rectum and anal canal.

The large intestine receives the fluid by-products of digestion from the ileocecal orifice or valve and slowly converts them to the more solid consistency of the feces preparatory to their excretion.

The cecum is that part of the large intestine beyond the attachment of the ileum. It is a blind pouch about 3 inches (7.5 cm) wide and long from the lower portion of which projects the vermiform appendix, average length about 3 inches (7.5 cm); its

function is unknown. At the opening of the ileum into the cecum is the ileocecal valve, a true sphincter, which controls the passage of the intestinal contents into the cecum.

The colon, which averages 4 to 6 feet in length (1.5 to 2 meters), is divided into ascending, transverse, descending and sigmoid portions. The ascending colon passes upward on the right of the abdomen from the cecum to the inferior surface of the liver, where it bends to become the transverse colon. This bend is called the right colic flexure. The transverse colon sweeps across the abdominal cavity from right to left, below the stomach. It is attached to the posterior abdominal wall by a peritoneal fold, the transverse mesocolon. At the spleen it bends downward to become the descending colon. This is the left colic flexure. The descending colon extends downward along the left side of the abdomen to the brim of the pelvis. From this point the colon courses in a curve like the letter "S" as far as the third segment of the sacrum, where it becomes the rectum. The S-shaped curve is called the sigmoid colon.

RECTAL AND ANAL CANAL

The rectum is about 5 inches (12 cm) long and continues from the sigmoid colon, at about the third sacral vertebrae, down to the pelvic diaphragm in front of the coccyx, where it joins the anal canal.

The anal canal, about 1 to 1 1/2 inches (3 cm) in length, is the terminal portion of the large intestine. The external aperture, called the anus, is guarded by an internal and external sphincter. It is kept closed except during defecation.

ABDOMINAL CAVITY

The abdominal cavity, the largest cavity in the body, contains the liver, stomach, intestines and the remaining portions of the digestive tract, and extends from the thorax to the floor of the pelvis.

The peritoneum, a thin, smooth, almost transparent serous membrane, lines the walls of the abdominal cavity as a parietal peritoneum and clothes varying areas of the viscera as visceral peritoneum. It is moistened with a lubricant serous fluid reducing friction between surfaces normally gliding and changing shape upon each other.

ACCESSORY ORGANS OF DIGESTION

Accessory organs of digestion are the salivary glands, liver, gallbladder and pancreas. The liver, gallbladder and pancreas are described below.

LIVER

The liver, the largest gland in the body, secretes bile and also receives digested carbohydrates and protein from the intestine by way of the portal vein. It fills the right upper portion of the abdominal cavity from the undersurface of the diaphragm to below the costal region. There is an extension to the left where it lies beneath the left cupola of the diaphragm and above the cardia of the stomach. The inferior vena cava is embedded in a deep groove on the back of the liver.

The liver has two principal lobes, the right and the left. The falciform ligament which passes from the liver to the diaphragm and the anterior abdominal wall forms the line of demarcation between the right and left lobes. The falciform ligament is a remnant of the anterior mesentery and conveys on its free border a fibrous cord, the occluded umbilical vein, now the round ligament. The surface of the liver is covered with peritoneum with the exception of a small area on its posterior surface that is attached directly to the diaphragm. Beneath the peritoneum is a dense connective tissue layer called the capsule of Glisson, which covers the entire surface of the organ, and at the hilum or porta is continued into the liver substance, forming a framework for the branches of the portal vein, hepatic artery and bile ducts.

The functions of the liver are described below to indicate the extent and versatility of this important organ.*

1. Formation of bile.
2. Activity of reticulo-endothelial tissues.
   (a) Hemopoiesis in the embryo

*Table from: Human Anatomy and Physiology. Barry G. King, Ph.D., and Mary Jane Showers, R.N., Ph.D., 5th Ed., W. B. Saunders Co. 1963.

   (b) Production of plasma proteins and antibodies
   (c) Destruction of red blood cells
   (d) Phagocytosis (Küpffer cells)
3. Metabolism of carbohydrates, lipids and proteins preparatory to use or excretion.
   (a) Glycogenesis, glycogenolysis, and gluconeogenesis to maintain normal blood sugar
   (b) Desaturation of fats and conversion of phospholipids
   (c) Synthesis of amino acids; formation of serum, albumin, serum globulin, antibodies, heparin, fibrinogen, and prothrombin
   (d) Deamination of amino acids; Conversion of protein to carbohydrates and fat
   (e) Formation of urea and uric acid; destruction of uric acid
4. Storage depot
   Glycogen
   Amino acids
   Fats
   Vitamins, A, D, B complex
   Iron and copper
5. Blood reservoir
6. Heat production
7. Detoxication
   Indol, skatol, phenol
   Morphine, strychnine, nicotine
   Steroid hormones
8. Formation of lymph

GALLBLADDER

The gallbladder is a pear-shaped, hollow sac attached to the under surface of the liver. It ends in the cystic duct, which joins with hepatic ducts to form the common bile duct. The gallbladder serves as a storage for the bile, which is secreted by the liver continuously. The bile may not immediately enter the intestines, but, after passing down the hepatic duct, may turn into the cystic duct and enter the gallbladder. The blood vessels and lymphatics absorb water and inorganic salts from the bile. At intervals during digestion, the gallbladder contracts and forces bile down the cystic duct and into the common bile duct, which opens into the duodenum about 10 cm below the pylorus. The common bile duct pierces the duodenal wall obliquely and joins with the pancreatic duct to form the Ampulla of Vater, which opens into the duodenum through a small elevation called the duodenal papilla. The orifice on the summit of the papilla is surrounded by muscle fibers that form a sphincter.

PANCREAS

The pancreas is a long, slender, vascular organ, with its head lying to the right in the loop of the duodenum, its body posterior to the stomach and its tail touching the spleen on the left. The pancreas is an important gland which secretes both an external secretion—pancreatic juice—important in digestion; and at least one internal secretion—insulin—concerned with carbohydrate metabolism.

Ducts from the lobules collect into a long pancreatic duct extending transversely from the tail to the head of the pancreas. At this point, the pancreatic duct is usually joined by an accessory pancreatic duct draining the head of the gland. The pancreatic duct empties into the duodenum with the common bile duct at the Ampulla of Vater. Scattered throughout the gland between the alveoli are groups of cells somewhat paler than the others which are called islets of Langerhans. They secrete insulin.

SURGICAL PROCEDURES— DIGESTIVE SYSTEM

Mouth

Incision
Drainage of sublingual abscess, e.g., under the tongue.
Drainage of Ludwig's angina, e.g., inflammation of the floor of the mouth and around the submaxillary gland.

Lips

Excision
V-excision of a lesion of a lip.
Resection of a lip lesion with or without plastic closure.
Repair
Cheiloplasty: Plastic or reconstruction operation on lip. Plastic repair of a harelip. Plastic repair of unilateral or bilateral harelip by re-creation of defect and reclosure.

Tongue

Incision
Glossotomy: Incision of tongue. Drainage of lingual abscess.
Excision
Glossectomy: Partial or complete excision of tongue. Biopsy of tongue.
Electrocoagulation: Coagulation of tissue by means of high frequency electric current.
Repair
Glossoplasty: Plastic operation on tongue.
Suture
Glossorrhaphy: Suture of tongue wound or injury.

Teeth and Gums

Incision
Drainage of alveolar abscess.

Palate and Uvula

Incision
Incision and drainage of palate for abscess.
Excision
Biopsy of palate.
Excision of local lesion of palate with graft or flap closure.
Resection of palate or wide excision of lesion of palate.
Resection of palate with reconstruction.
Uvulectomy: Excision of uvula.
Repair
Palatoplasty: Plastic operation of partial cleft palate for complete cleft palate, including alveolar ridge, major revision, secondary lengthening procedure or attachment of pharyngeal flap.
Suture
Suture palate wound or injury.

Salivary Glands and Ducts

Incision
Drainage of a parotid abscess.
Sialolithotomy: Removal of a calculus from a salivary gland or duct.
Excision
Biopsy of a salivary gland.
Excision of a parotid tumor.

Repair

Sialodochoplasty: Plastic repair of a salivary duct.

Suture

Closure of a salivary fistula.

Manipulation

Ptyalectasis: Dilation of a salivary duct.

Pharynx, Adenoids and Tonsils

Incision

Drainage of retropharyngeal abscess, internal or external approach.

Drainage of peritonsillar abscess.

Biopsy of the pharynx.

Excision

Pharyngectomy: Surgical excision of a part of the pharynx.

Adenoidectomy: Excision of the adenoids.

Tonsillectomy: Excision of the tonsils.

Repair

Pharyngoplasty: Plastic operation on the pharynx.

Suture

Suture of external wound or injury of the pharynx.

Esophagus

Incision

Esophagotomy: An incision into the esophagus.

Esophagostomy: Surgical creation of an artificial opening into the esophagus.

Esophagogastrostomy: Formation of a communication between the esophagus and stomach.

Excision

Esophagectomy: Excision of part of the esophagus.

Esophagogastrectomy: Excision of esophagus and stomach.

Endoscopy

Examination of the esophagus by the use of an esophagoscope.

Esophagoscopy: Diagnostic.

Repair

Esophagoplasty: Plastic repair or reconstruction of the esophagus.

Esophagogastrostomy: Forming an artificial communication between the esophagus and stomach.

Esophagostomy: Forming an artificial opening into the esophagus.

Esophagoduodenostomy: Surgical anastomosis between the esophagus and the duodenum.

Esophago-enterostomy: Suturing the esophagus to the jejunum and usually excising the stomach.

Esophagogastroplasty: Plastic repair of the esophagus and stomach.

Esophagojejunogastrostomosis: Mobilizing a loop of jejunum and implanting its proximal end in the esophagus and its distal end in the stomach.

Esophagojejunostomy: Surgical anastomosis between the esophagus and the jejunum.

Suture

Suture of esophageal wound, injury or rupture, via cervical approach.

Stomach

Incision

Gastrotomy: Surgical incision into the stomach.

Gastrostomy: Surgical creation of a gastric fistula.

Pyloromyotomy: Longitudinal incision of the circular muscles of the pylorus (Ramstedt operation).

Pylorotomy: Surgical incision of the pylorus.

Laparotomy: Surgical opening of the abdomen.

Excision

Gastrectomy: Surgical removal of a part, or the whole of the stomach.

Pylorogastrectomy: Excision of the pyloric portion of the stomach.

Gastropylorectomy: Excision of the pyloric portion of the stomach.

Antrectomy with total gastric or selective vagotomy.

Repair

Gastrocolostomy: Surgical creation of an artificial passage from the stomach to the colon (accidental).

Gastroenteocolostomy: Surgical creation of an artificial passage between the stomach, intestines and colon (accidental).

Gastroduodenostomy: Surgical creation of an anastomosis between the stomach and duodenum.

Gastroenterostomy: Surgical creation of an anastomosis between the stomach and small bowel.

Suture

Pyloroplasty: Surgical repair of the pylorus to increase its aperture by enlarging the pyloric opening from the stomach.

Gastrorrhaphy: Suturing of a wound of the stomach.

Endoscopy

Gastroscopy: Diagnostic, or with biopsy.

Intestines

Incision

Gastroenterotomy: Surgical incision of stomach and intestines.

Enterotomy: Incision for dissection of the intestines.

Enterostomy: Surgical formation of an opening into the intestine through the abdominal wall.

Excision

Enterectomy: Surgical excision of a part of the intestine; resection of the intestine.

Repair

Enterocholecystostomy: Surgical formation of an opening from the gallbladder to the small intestine.

Enterocolostomy: Surgical formation of a communication between the small intestine and the colon.

Enterostomy: Surgical formation of a permanent opening into the intestine through the abdominal wall.

Enteroplasty: Plastic surgery of the intestine, for enlargement of a constricted bowel.

Ileocolostomy: Surgical formation of a permanent opening between the ileum and colon (usually transverse colon).

Suture

Enterorrhaphy: The act of suturing a wound of the intestine.

Meckel's Diverticulum and Mesentery

Excision

Meckel's diverticulectomy: Excision

of a Meckel's diverticulum.

Suture

Mesentorrhaphy: Operation of suturing the mesentery (the peritoneal fold attaching the intestine to the posterior abdominal wall).

Cecum and Colon

Incision

Cecotomy: Surgical incision into the cecum.

Colopexotomy: Surgical fixation and incision of the colon.

Colotomy: Surgical incision into the colon.

Excision

Celiectomy: Surgical removal of any abdominal organ.

Cecectomy: Surgical removal of a part of the cecum.

Repair

Colostomy: Surgical formation of a permanent opening into the colon through the abdominal wall.

Cecostomy: Surgical formation of a permanent opening into the cecum through the abdominal wall.

Sigmoidostomy: Surgical formation of a permanent opening into the sigmoid colon through the abdominal wall.

Cecocolostomy: Surgical formation of an anastomosis between the cecum and the colon.

Cecosigmoidostomy: Surgical formation of an anastomosis between the cecum and the sigmoid.

Colopexostomy: Resection of the colon with cecostomy or appendicostomy.

Colorectostomy: Surgical formation of a new passage between the colon and the rectum.

Suture

Colorrhaphy: Surgical suturing of the colon.

Appendix

Excision

Appendectomy: Surgical removal of the vermiform appendix.

Repair

Appendicostomy: Surgical formation of a permanent opening into the appendix through the abdominal wall.

Rectum (Procto-, proct-) and Anus

Incision

Rectostomy: Surgical creation of an artificial opening into rectum for stricture.

Proctovalvotomy: Surgical incision of the rectal valves.

Proctotomy: Surgical opening of an imperforate anus.

Repair

Proctocystotomy: Rectovesical operation for stone in the bladder.

Proctoperineoplasty: Plastic repair of the anus and perineum.

Proctopexy: Surgical fixation of the rectum to another part by suture.

Proctoplasty: Plastic surgery of the anus and rectum.

Proctostomy: Surgical creation of a permanent opening into the rectum.

Excision

Proctosigmoidectomy: Surgical excision of the anus and sigmoid flexure.

Suture

Proctorrhaphy: Plastic suture of the rectum.

Liver (Hepato-, hepat- hepatico-)

Incision

Hepaticolithotomy: Surgical incision of the hepatic duct.

Hepaticotomy: Surgical incision of the hepatic duct.

Hepatotomy: Surgical incision of the liver.

Excision

Hepatectomy: Surgical excision of a portion of the liver; or excision of a lesion of the liver.

Repair

Hepaticocholangiocholecystenterostomy: The formation of a communication between the gallbladder and a hepatic duct and between the intestine and the gallbladder.

Hepaticocholangiojejunostomy: The formation of a communication between the gallbladder, a hepatic duct, and the jejunum.

Hepaticoduodenostomy: The formation of a communication between a hepatic duct and the duodenum.

Hepatico-gastrostomy: The creation of a communication between a hepatic duct and the stomach.

Hepaticojejunostomy: The creation of an opening between a hepatic duct and the jejunum.

Hepatocholangiocystoduodenostomy: A surgical procedure to establish drainage of the bile ducts into the duodenum via the gallbladder.

Hepatocholangioduodenostomy: A surgical operation to establish drainage of the bile ducts into the duodenum.

Hepatocholangiogastrostomy: A surgical procedure to establish drainage of the bile ducts into the stomach.

Hepatocholangioenterostomy: Surgical formation of a communication between the liver and the intestine.

Hepatocholangiostomy: A surgical procedure to establish drainage of the gallbladder either through the abdominal wall or by means of internal drainage into some part of the gastrointestinal tract.

Hepatoduodenostomy: The formation of a communication between the liver and the duodenum.

Abdomen, Peritoneum and Omentum

Endoscopy

Peritoneoscopy: A telescopic instrument for examination of the perineal cavity.

Introduction

Pneumoperitoneum: Intraperitoneal injection of air; retroperitoneal insufflation of air.

Repair

Perineoplasty: Repair on the perineum.

Herniaplasty, Herniorrhaphy, Herniotomy

Inguinal, unilateral; with appendectomy; with orchiectomy; with excision or hydrocele or recurrent. Inguinal, bilateral; recurrent direct or indirect.

Femoral, unilateral; with appendectomy, recurrent.

Femoral, bilateral; recurrent.

Ventral, incisional; recurrent.

Epigastric, recurrent.

Umbilical.

Omphalocele.

Diaphragmatic.

Suture

    Hepatorrhaphy: Suture repair of a liver laceration.

Gallbladder
(Chole-, chol-, cholo-)

Incision

    Cholangiotomy: Surgical incision of an intrahepatic duct for removal of gallstones

    Cholecystostomy: Surgical incision into the gallbladder with drainage.

    Cholecystotomy: Surgical incision of the gallbladder.

    Choledochotomy: Surgical incision of the common bile duct.

    Cholelithotomy: Surgical removal of gallstones by means of an incision.

Excision

    Choledochectomy: Surgical excision of a portion of the common duct for carcinoma of the bile duct.

    Cholecystectomy: Surgical removal of the gallbladder.

Suture

    Cholecystorrhaphy: Suturation of the gallbladder.

    Choledochorrhaphy: Surgical procedure of suturing the incised common bile duct.

Repair

    Cholecystocolostomy: The formation of a passage from the gallbladder to the colon.

    Cholecystoduodenostomy: A surgical formation of a communication between the gallbladder and the duodenum.

    Cholecystogastrostomy: A surgical formation of a communication between the gallbladder and the stomach.

    Cholecysto-ileostomy: Formation of an opening between the gallbladder and the ileum.

    Cholecystojejunostomy: The formation of a communication between the gallbladder and the jejunum.

    Cholecystopyelostomy: The surgical formation of a communication of the gallbladder with the pelvis of the kidney.

    Choledochocholedocostomy: The formation of a communication between two portions of the common bile duct.

    Choledochoduodenostomy: The formation of an opening between the common bile duct and the duodenum.

    Choledocho-enterostomy: The creation of a passage from the common bile duct to the intestine.

    Choledochogastrostomy: The formation of a communication between the common bile duct and the stomach.

    Choledocho-jejunostomy: The formation of a communication between the common bile duct and the jejunum.

    Choledochostomy: The surgical formation of an opening into the common bile duct.

    Choledochoplasty: The surgical operation on the common bile duct, as for biliary fistula.

Pancreas

Incision

    Pancreatolithotomy: Surgical incision of the pancreas for the removal of calculus.

    Pancreatotomy: Surgical incision of the pancreas.

    Pancreolithotomy: Surgical incision into the pancreas for the removal of calculus.

Excision

    Pancreatectomy: Surgical removal of all or part of the pancreas.

    Pancreatoduodenectomy: Excision of the head of the pancreas along with the encircling loop of the duodenum.

    Pancreatolithotomy: Excision of a calculus from the pancreas.

Repair

    Pancreaticoduodenostomy: Surgical anastomosis of the pancreatic duct and the duodenum.

    Pancreatico-enterostomy: Surgical communication of the pancreatic duct and the intestine.

    Pancreaticogastrostomy: Implantation of the cut end of the pancreas into the wall of the stomach after excision of part of the pancreas.

    Pancreaticojejunostomy: Communication of the pancreatic duct and the jejunum.

ENDOCRINE SYSTEM

There should be no schism in the body . . . the members should have the same care one for another. I CORINTHIANS 12, 25

The endocrine glands have no ducts, and hence are often referred to as the ductless glands or glands of internal secretion because their secretions are poured directly into the blood stream. The secretions of the endocrine group control the orderly functioning of the body; some are essential for life itself. The active principles of the endocrine glands are called hormones, from a Greek word meaning "I stimulate." However, their substances can inhibit as well as stimulate.

The endocrine system is composed of a number of glands that play a major role supplementing the effect of the nervous system in regulating the rate of various physiological processes and maintaining the constancy of the internal environment of the body. The endocrine glands are shown in Plate 36.

The endocrine glands may be divided into three groups: (1) the pituitary (hypophysis cerebri); (2) the thyroid, suprarenal and reproductive glands (ovaries and testes), which are under the control of the pituitary; and (3) the parathyroid glands, pancreas, placenta and gastrointestinal mucosa, which are independent of pituitary control.

PITUITARY GLAND OR HYPOPHYSIS CEREBRI

The human pituitary gland is a small organ, rounded and approximately half an inch in diameter, hangs by its stalk or infundibulum from the tuber cinereum of the floor of the third ventricle. It lies in the sella turcica of the sphenoid bone below the optic chiasma. Posteriorly it is bounded by a plate of bone, the dorsum sellae, from the upper lateral margins of which the posterior clinoid processes project anteriorly. The anterior wall of the sella turcica terminates above in the tuberculum sellae, on either side of which are seen membrane which is continuous with the dura covering the floor of the skull. It is attached to the dorsum sellae behind, the tuberculum sellae in front

and to strong interclinoid ligaments laterally, which stretch from the posterior to the anterior clinoid processes. The roof is perforated by a foramen through which the infundibulum passes to the floor of the third ventricle. The lateral walls of the sella turcica are membranous and are formed by the medial walls of the cavernous sinuses; the floor is bony and immediately beneath it lies the sphenoid sinus.

The pituitary gland arises from two sources, epithelial and neural ectoderm. The pituitary gland is regarded as a regulating organ controlling primarily the other endocrine glands and having perhaps some metabolic functions of its own. It is a marvel that such a small gland as this almost rules the whole of the body. Barger called it the "general headquarters" of the endocrine system and Cushing even more picturesquely, the "leader of the endocrine orchestra." However, today this pituitary gland deserves the title of "conductor," being the only gland to produce hormones that specifically affect other glands, i.e., the (target glands) thyroid, adrenals and gonads. If a target gland cannot produce enough of its own hormone to supply the body's needs, the pituitary thus stimulated will produce or secrete a larger amount of the particular hormone, an interrelationship known as a feedback system.

Thus, the "endocrine orchestra" is affected by temperature (cold affects the function of the thyroid); the egg-laying cycle of chickens can be regulated by altering the duration and color of light. (Glandular secretions are influenced by race, sex, season and diet.) The glands maintaining an intricate feedback among themselves, together with their surrounding tissues, are in turn enmeshed in a larger network which includes the nervous system. It is believed that the hypothalamus, under the control of the brain, exercises a control over the pituitary and thus through that gland over the entire endocrine system. Therefore, emerging from the belief that the pituitary gland was the conductor of the endocrine orchestra, it now appears that the pituitary is just the concert master receiving directions from a higher cerebral conductor. The best known mechanism is that of fear; a psychic impulse stimulates the production of adrenaline, which in turn stimulates the pituitary, thyroid and pancreas.

The anterior lobe of the pituitary is the vital part since destruction of the posterior lobe alone leads only to a disturbance of water metabolism.

Pituitary insufficiency is produced by a variety of destructive lesions of the anterior lobe of the pituitary gland, and results in atrophy of the other endocrine organs under its control. During adult life it causes Simmonds' disease in which are combined many of the symptoms of deficiency of the atrophied endocrine glands. During childhood and adolescence it also delays growth and causes pituitary dwarfism. A congenital pituitary insufficiency results in a form of pituitary dwarfism called ateleiosis.

Six anterior pituitary hormones have been obtained as homogeneous or almost homogeneous proteins; they are the two gonadotrophic, the lactogenic, the corticotrophic, the thyrotrophic and the growth hormones.

The hormones of the posterior lobe stimulate the smooth muscle of the uterus and blood vessels and assist in regulating the water balance of the body. Damage to this lobe or its connections with the brain causes diabetes insipidus, excess secretion of dilute urine.

SUPRARENAL GLANDS

The suprarenal glands are a pair of flattened, yellowish organs about 2 inches high, 1 inch wide and $1/2$ inch thick, situated posteriorly in the abdomen behind the peritoneum on either side of the spine and immediately above and in front of the upper poles of the kidneys. They are also called adrenal glands, both names meaning "above the kidney."

They are surrounded by areolar tissue containing a considerable amount of fat. The right gland is somewhat pyramidal and the left is semilunar, usually larger and situated a little higher than the right. The

average weight of each in the adult is from 3 to 4 g. Each organ is closely invested by a connective-tissue capsule which may contain muscle fibers. Trabeculae pass from the capsule into the substance of the gland.

There is a rich blood supply to the suprarenal glands derived from the aorta, and the inferior phrenic and renal arteries.

In structure, function and also development, the gland comprises two organs, a yellow, convoluted, $1/4$-inch thick cortex, surrounding a thinner reddish-grey medulla. The cortex, which also gives origin to the sex glands, secretes hormones concerned with bodily strength and sex development. Before puberty the cortex increases rapidly and middle age marks the onset of atrophy. The medulla secretes adrenalin, which boosts the effect of the sympathetic system in violent effort for flight or fight as the occasion demands.

THYROID GLAND

The thyroid gland is a horseshoe-shaped organ with two lateral lobes and an isthmus. It weighs in an adult about 25 to 30 g. but variations occur with age, sex, body weight, stature and climate. It lies in the front and sides of the neck at the level of the fifth, sixth and seventh cervical vertebrae. The gland is highly vascular.

The known functions of the thyroid are three: (1) the concentration of iodine; (2) the conversion of iodine into the thyroid hormone; and (3) the release of the hormone into the circulation. The thyroid hormone controls the rate of cellular metabolism in all tissues of the body. The activity of the thyroid is chiefly controlled by the thyrotrophic hormone of the anterior pituitary.

The secretion of the thyroid gland is called thyroxin, a hormone which is vital for growth and metabolism. Enlargement of the gland is seen in youth, and in women during menstruation and pregnancy.

PARATHYROID GLANDS

These glands are small, yellowish-brown bodies usually located on the posterior surface of each thyroid lobe near its medial border. They may be implanted in the thyroid gland or behind the pharynx or even in the thorax with the thymus. Most individuals have two pairs.

The parathyroids are concerned with the regulation of the calcium and phosphate metabolism of the body and are essential to life. Excess secretion, hyperparathyroidism from parathyroid tumors, causes the calcium of the skeleton to be carried away in the blood, the bones becoming light, porous and brittle. The parathyroid glands secrete parathormone.

THYMUS

The two lobes (a soft pink, glandular mass) of the thymus occupy the upper mediastinum and lower part of the neck, e.g., the mass in the root of the neck and upper part of the thorax extending from the lower border of the thyroid gland to the level of the fourth costal cartilages. They lie beneath the manubrium sterni and the sternohyoid and sternothyroid muscles. The pleura overlaps the lower poles of the lobes. Behind lies the trachea, the left innominate and inferior thyroid veins and the aortic arch, the innominate and left common carotid arteries, the phrenic, vagus and recurrent laryngeal nerves. The blood supply is provided by the internal mammary superior and inferior thyroid arteries. The vagus and sympathetic nerves send branches to the gland.

In structure the thymus consists of lobules bound together by connective tissue which forms a thin capsule for the whole gland; however, it retains the secret of its function though it is believed to be associated with muscle activity.

PANCREAS

The pancreas is an organ that extends transversely across the posterior abdominal wall from the duodenal loop on the right to the hilus of the spleen on the left. This gland contains both exocrine and endocrine tissue. Here we are concerned with the endocrine tissue, called the islets of Langerhans, consisting of two types of cells, alpha (α) cells and beta (β) cells—the α cells secrete the hormone glucagon and the β cells secrete insulin.

Insulin is essential to life; if deficient, hyperglycemia (elevated blood glucose)

and consequently glycosuria (glucose in urine) develop. This condition is known as *diabetes mellitus.*

GONADS

The testes and ovaries in addition to forming the male and female reproductive cells also secrete into the blood stream certain substances which control the appearance of secondary sex characteristics.

PLACENTA

The placenta is an organ developed within the uterus during pregnancy in order that the growing fetus may secure nourishment from the maternal blood stream and may excrete its waste material into the maternal blood. Certain cells of the placenta are known to be a source of sex hormones, and it is, therefore, a temporary gland of the endocrine system.

PINEAL BODY

The pineal body is a small cone-shaped mass of tissue, about 1/4 inch in length, attached by means of a hollow stalk to the roof of the third ventricle of the brain and lying on the superior colliculi. Although classified with the ductless glands, its function is unknown, but in the present state of our knowledge, it is mainly important clinically in the showing by the 18th year calcareous granules; the displacement of these granules to one side in X-rays indicates the presence of a tumor on the opposite side.

INTERNAL SECRETIONS OF GASTRIC AND INTESTINAL MUCOSA

Hormones are but one factor in the complex chemical system of the body fluids controlling physiological integration, health, development and behavior.

Gastrin is a hormone secreted into the blood by the mucous membrane lining of the pyloric or antrum end of the stomach, carried by the blood to the chief and parietal cells of the fundus and body of the stomach (see P. 78), which it stimulates to secrete pepsin and acid, respectively. The duodenum contains cells which secrete prosecretin, which remains inactive until the medium is acidified. When the acid chyme from the stomach enters the duodenum, prosecretin is released, changed to secretin, absorbed by the blood and carried to the pancreas, liver and intestines, thus stimulating each organ to secretory activity.

TABLE II

*Endocrine glands with commonly used synonyms and their secretion**

Gland	Synonym	Secretion
Hypophis cerebri	Pituitary gland	
Pars distalis	Anterior pituitary	ACTH, TSH, FSH, LTH,
Pars tuberalis		ICSH, STH
Pars intermedia	Intermediate lobe of pituitary	Intermedin
Pars nervosa	Posterior pituitary	ADH (vasopressin) and Oxytocin
Thyroid	None	Thyroxin and Triiodothyronine
Parathyroids	None	Parathorimone
Pancreas	None	
Islets of Langerhans	Pancreatic islets	α-cells, glucagon; β-cells, insulin
Suprarenals	Adrenal glands	
Cortex	Adrenal cortex	Cortisone, hydrocortisone and aldosterone
Medulla	Adrenal medulla	Epinephrine and norepinephrine
Ovaries	None	
Thecal cells	Theca interna	Estradiol, estriol, and estrone
Corpus lutea		Progesterone
Testes	None	
Interstitial cells	Leydig cells	Androgens, mainly testosterone

*From King, B. G., and Showers, M.J.: *Human Physiology and Anatomy*, ed. 5. W.B. Saunders Company, Philadelphia, 1963.

SURGICAL PROCEDURES— ENDOCRINE SYSTEM

Thyroid Gland

Incision

Thyrochondrotomy: Surgical incision of the thyroid cartilage.

Thyrocricotomy: Tracheotomy through the cricothyroid membrane.

Thyrofissure: Surgical creation of an opening through the thyroid cartilage to gain access to the interior of the larynx.

Thyroidotomy: Surgical incision of the thyroid. Incision and drainage of thyroglossal cyst (infected).

Exicsion

Thyroidectomy: Surgical excision of the thyroid.

Thyroparathyroidectomy: Excision of the thyroid and parathyroids. Local excision of small cyst or adenoma of thyroid.

Parathyroid, Thymus, Pituitary, Pineal, Adrenal Glands and Carotid Bodies

Excision

Parathyroidectomy: Excision of a parathyroid.

Adrenalectomy: Excision of the adrenal glands, unilateral or bilateral.

Ovariectomy: Excision of the ovaries, unilateral or bilateral.

Pinealectomy: Excision of the pineal body.

Mediastinal exploration.

Excision of carotid body tumor.

Glomectomy: Excision of a carotid body.

Hypophysectomy: Surgical removal of the hypophysis, or pituitary gland.

SENSORY SYSTEM

If the whole body were an eye, where were the hearing? . . . . If the whole body were hearing, where were the smelling? I CORINTHIANS 12, 17

The organs of special sense enhance the faculty by which the conditions of things are perceived: hearing and equilibrium; vision, smell and taste; varieties of sense, hunger, thirst and malaise; and those associated with the general sensations of temperature, time, pain and pressure; and, of course, our well-being.

The sensory unit includes (1) a peripheral end organ, or receptor, (2) the sensory path through which the impulses are conveyed, and (3) a center in the cortex which interprets the sensation. It is through the sensory units that man derives information about himself and the world in which he lives. Sensations are the conscious results of processes which take place within the brain in consequence of nervous impulses derived from receptors. A number of sensations are not followed by motor reactions but are stored as memory concepts to be used when needed.

EAR

The ear is concerned with the functions of hearing and equilibrium. The ear consists of three divisions, external, middle, and internal, with the greater part of it being enclosed in the temporal bone. The middle ear is in direct communication with the nose and throat. The internal ear contains the sensory organs for perception of sound (acoustic labyrinth) and the maintenance of body equilibrium (static and kinetic labyrinth); the former constituting the cochlea portion and the latter the vestibular portion.

EXTERNAL EAR

The *external ear* (Plate 37) is that portion of the auditory apparatus situated laterally to the tympanic membrane (ear drum) which consists of the auricle (pinna) and the external auditory meatus or canal, a little over an inch in length, which leads from the external ear to the middle ear. The auricle is an irregularly shaped plate of cartilaginous framework covered with skin projecting from each side of the head and serves to collect and direct sound waves into the external acoustic meatus. The auricle consists of: (1) helix (2) antihelix (3) crus of helix (4) tragus (5) concha (6) antitragus (7) lobule (8) external auditory meatus and (9) Darwin's tubercle.

The cartilage of the pinna is continuous with that of the external canal in front and below, forming an incomplete tube open above and anteriorly, where it is joined by a tough fibrous tissue membrane extending between the tragus and the commencement of the helix. The helix is the circular, folded, outer edge of the pinna; the antihelix is the smaller ridge just opposite it. The tragus is the small, tongue-like projection anterior to the meatus. The lobule is composed of adipose and connective tissue.

The canal is lined with skin which presents many fine hairs and sebaceous glands near its orifice. Along the upper wall are the ceruminous glands, modified sweat glands that secrete the ear wax or cerumen. The hairs and cerumen help to prevent the entrance of foreign particles into the ear.

MIDDLE EAR

The middle ear contains the mechanism for the conduction of air-borne sound waves to the internal ear. Described best as a six-sided box, 15 mm in length from above downward and from behind forward, very narrow from side to side, and wider above and deeper behind than in front.

The middle ear or tympanic cavity, is a small, irregular bony cavity situated in the petrous portion of the temporal bone. The eustachian tube connects the middle ear and the nasopharynx thus providing an air passage which equalizes pressure on both sides of the ear drum. By this means air pressure within the cavity is equalized with that outside. Equalization of pressure is aided by swallowing. The Eustacian tube normally is closed. Through the posterior wall is an opening into the mastoid antrum and mastoid cells. Two openings covered with membrane (the round and oval windows) separate the cavity from the inner ear. A chain of three small bones (the ossicles) extends across the cavity from the tympanic membrane to the oval window, the hammer (malleus), anvil (incus) and stirrup (stapes). The malleus is attached to the drum membrane; the stapes fit into the oval window. Vibrations set up in the tympanic membrane by sound waves reaching it through the auditory meatus are transmitted to the inner ear through the ossicles which bridge the cavity.

INNER EAR

The internal ear (Plate 37) contains the essential organs for hearing and equilibrium. It consists of bony and membranous portions. The bony part is called the osseous labyrinth, composed of a series of canals named from their shape: (1) the vestibule, which occupies a central position between the cochlea in front and the semicircular canals behind; (2) the cochlea (snail shell); and (3) the semicircular canals tunneled out in the petrous portion of the temporal bone. The membranous labyrinth lies within the osseous labyrinth. The former is filled with a liquid called endolymph and the latter perilymph.

SURGICAL PROCEDURES—EAR

External Ear

Incision

Ototomy: Surgical incision into, or dissection of the ear (anatomy).

Drainage of abscess of auricle.

Drainage of hemotoma of auricle.

Drainage of abscess of external auditory canal.

Excision

Biopsy of ear.

Local destruction of lesion of ear with plastic closure.

Otonecrectomy; Otonecronectomy: Excision of necrosed tissues from the ear.

Excision of exostosis of external auditory canal.

Otoscleronectomy: Surgical excision of sclerosed and ankylosed ear ossicles.

Repair

Otoplasty: Plastic surgery (reparative) of the auricle of the ear.

Reconstruction of ear with graft or skin plus cartilage, bone or other implant.

Otoplasty, of cartilage ("lop ear") with or without reduction in size.

Middle Ear

Incision

Ossiculotomy: Division of one of the processes of the ossicles of the middle ear.

Eustachian tube, catheterization and insufflation.

Myringotomy: Incision of the tympanic membrane.

Tympanotomy: Incision of the membrana tympani.

Plicotomy: Surgical cutting of the posterior fold of the tympanic membrane.

Mastoidotomy: Incision into mastoid process of the temporal bone.

Excision

Myringectomy: Excision of the tympanic membrane.

Mastoidectomy (Simple or radical): Hollowing out of the mastoid process by excising the bony partitions which form the mastoid cells.

Stapedectomy: Excision of stapes in the ear.

Removal of middle ear polyp by snare.

Ossiculectomy: Excision of an ossicle or bonelet, particularly one of the bones of the tympanum.

Myringodectomy: Excision of tympanum.

Tympanectomy: Excision of the tympanic membrane.

Repair

Tympanoplasty (may include complete mastoidectomy): Surgical correction of a damaged middle ear.

Myringoplasty: Plastic operation to repair a damaged tympanic membrane.

Reconstruction of canal and middle ear for agenesis (congenital atresis of ear canal).

Mastoideocentesis: Surgical puncture of the mastoid process.

Internal Ear

Incision

Labyrinthotomy: Incision of the labyrinth.

Excision

Labyrinthectomy: Excision of the labyrinth.

Repair

Fenestration of seimcircular canals: Formation of an artificial opening into labyrinth of the ear.

Stapes mobilization: to relieve conductive hearing impairment resulting from its immobilization through disease.

EYE

The eye (Plate 38) is referred to as "the light of the body," which is quite true, for in addition to vision, many problems are reflected. Through observation with an ophthalmoscope and thorough examination of the eye, early warnings of diabetes, high blood pressure (hypertension), jaundice, anemia, certain tumors, allergies and other disorders are revealed.

Similar to a camera, some of the structures of the eye form sharp images. Other structures, similar to the film of a camera, react to light rays composing the image, setting up the nerve impulses which give rise to the sensations of form, contrast and color by which the objects are recognized.

The associated structures which protect the eye and aid in its function are the orbital cavities, the eyelids, the lacrimal apparatus and the eye muscles.

The skin of the eyelids is the thinnest in the body, very elastic and recovers rapidly after distention with fluid. Skin of the medial half of the eyelids is greasy—unicellular with many sebaceous glands; its lateral half is less greasy and contains a large number of hairs which are attached to medial and lateral palpebral ligaments.

The eye is the paramount sense organ of the body detecting the first threat of danger; in reality a window viewing the world, it discerns thousands of diamond-shaped sunbeams dancing on a lake, reveling in the beauty of the transcient hues of a distant rainbow.

Slightly flattened from above downwards, the eyeball is so nearly spherical that anterior and posterior poles, meridians through the poles as an equator, are discovered.

Its walls are formed of three layers: an outer fibrous coat, a middle vascular coat, and an inner nervous coat. The fibrous coat has two parts, the sclera and the cornea. The sclera is tough and opaque and gives form to the eyeball. The cornea is the clear, transparent tissue that completes this coat anteriorly. The cornea is, however, more convex than the rest, and across its base the cavity of the eye is partially divided by a diaphragm, the iris. The cornea and lens of the eye focus the light upon the back or fundus of the eyeball, formed from without inwards by the protective sclera, the nutritive choroid and the sensory retina.

The vascular coat has many blood vessels and is concerned chiefly with nutrition of the eye. There are four parts of this vascular coat. (1) The choroid, which contains a rich plexus of blood vessels and a large amount of dark brown pigment, which reduces reflection and scattering of light after it has fallen on the retina, and is continuous with the ciliary body in front. (2) The ciliary muscles and ciliary process make up the ciliary body, which projects into the cavity of the eye at the sclerocorneal junction to form a circular band. (3) The iris, or colored portion of the eye, is a muscular diaphragm that is attached at its circumference to the ciliary body and has an opening, the pupil in the center. It controls the amount of light admitted to the eye. Its circular fibers, when stimulated, produce constriction of the pupil; its radial fibers contract to dilate the pupil. (4) The nervous coat or retina forms the lining layer of the eyeball. It contains rods and cones which are specialized cells sensitive to light rays, and these rods and cones are connected with the optic nerve.

The optic nerve leaves the eye slightly to the nasal side of center; the point is marked by a white circular area called the optic disc. Since there are no rods or cones in this area it is called the blind spot, because light rays focused on the ensheathed nerve cannot be seen. A few millimeters lateral to the optic disc and directly behind the pupil is a small yellow area called the macula lutea containing a central depression, the fovea centralis. This is the region of keenest vision.

The crystalline lens lies just behind the pupil and iris, held in position by the sensory ligaments, which are attached to the ciliary process. The iris separates the anterior and posterior chambers. The posterior chamber is the small recess between the iris in front and the suspensory ligament behind. Posterior to the lens is the large cavity of the eye filled with a jelly-like material called the vitreous humor. The aqueous humor fills the space anterior to the lens.

SURGICAL PROCEDURES—EYE

Eyeball

Incision

Goniotomy: Surgical opening of Schlemm's canal (*sinus venosus sclerae*) via the angle of the anterior chamber.

Cornea

Incision

Keratotomy: Surgical incision through the cornea.

Paracentesis of cornea (keratocentesis): Tapping: by passage into a cavity of a trocar or cannula for the purpose of removing fluid; An opening of the anterior chamber for the purpose of evacuating its contents (partially or completely; also done to reduce the raised intraocular pressure.

Excision

Keratectomy: Excision of a portion of the cornea; (partial superficial or total superficial).

Introduction

Curettage and cauterization of corneal ulcer.

Ionotophoresis of corneal ulcer.

Repair

Keratoplasty: Plastic operation on the cornea.

Corneal transplantation; Trephining of the cornea.

Corneal grafting—full thickness graft, or partial thickness (Lamella) graft.

Corneo-conjunctivoplasty: Surgical repair of cornea and conjunctiva.

Tattooing: Cornea—cosmetic procedure.

Suture

Suture of a perforated cornea.

Sclera

Incision

Sclerostomy: Formation of an opening in the sclera.

Scleroticotomy: Surgical incision of scleratic coat of the eye.

Excision

Sclerectomy: Excision of a part of the sclera.

Iris and Ciliary Body

Incision

Iridotomy (corectomy): Division of part of the iris; cutting of the iris.

Iridotomy (sphincterotomy): Transverse division of the fibers of the iris; forming an artificial pupil.

Iridosclerotomy: Incision of both the iris and sclera.

Synechiotomy: Division of the adhesion in synechia.

Cyclotomy: Surgical incision of the ciliary muscle.

Excision

Iridectomesodialysis: Surgical formation of an artificial pupil by separating adhesions around the inner margin of the iris.

Iridectomy: (also peripheral or capsulo-): Removal of a portion of the iris.

Iridocyclectomy: Removal of the iris and ciliary body.

Iris sphincterectomy: Excision of a portion of the pupillary border of the iris, to facilitate extraction of a cataract.

Pupillotomy: By light coagulation.

Cyclectomy: Excision of a portion of the ciliary muscle or body (also ciliary border of eyelid), (partial).

Iris Bombe': Surgical procedure to transfix the bombe' part of the iris where it is separated from the lens capsule due to an accumulation of aqueous in the posterior chamber.

Cyclodialysis: Establishment of a communication between the anterior chamber and suprachorioidal space.

Destruction

Cyclodiathermy: Destruction of the ciliary body by diathermy.

Cycloanemization: Obstruction of the long ciliary arteries in the surgical treatment of glaucoma.

Corelysis: Loosening of adhesions between the capsule of the lens and the iris.

Diathermy circumvallation: Destruction by electro-desiccation with a fine diathermy needle.

Manipulation

Iridencleisis: Incarceration of a portion of the iris to effect a displacement of the pupil.

Repair

Coreoplasty: Reestablishment of an occluded/or correction of, a deformed pupil.

Crystalline Lens

Incision

Discission: Incision or cutting through a part, and breaking up the substance of a crystalline lens.

Capsulotomy: Incision through capsule of the lens in a cataract operation.

Excision

Erisiphake extraction: The removal of a lens by suction.

Extraction of lens: Intracapsular: (a) immature cataract, (b) hypermature cataract, (c) dislocated lens. Extracapsular: (a) Forward bulging of the iris, (b) Complicated cataract, (c) High myopia, and (d) Cataract nigra.

Sclera

Incision

Sclerotomy: Incision through the sclerotic coat of the eye.

Anterior sclerotomy: Cutting a small three-sided "trap-door" of sclera hinged at the limbus.

Posterior sclerotomy: Incision through the sclera into the vitreous humor.

Excision

Sclerectomy: Removal of a part of the sclera.

Sclerectoiridectomy: Combination sclerectomy and iridectomy to form a filtering cicatrix.

Cornea

Incision

Peritomy: Dividing blood vessels extending abnormally from the limbus to the superficial layers of the cornea; Removal of a paracorneal strip of the conjunctiva.

Excision

Keratectomy: Excision of a portion of

the cornea. (partial superficial) or (total superficial).

Repair

Keratoplasty: Trephining of the cornea; corneal transplantation; Full-thickness corneal graft; partial thickness (Lamella) corneal graft.

Vitreous

Vitreous implant and replacement

Retina

Repair

Reattachment of retina, electrocoagulation.

Examination

Funduscopic, under anesthesia.

Ocular Muscles

Recession and Resection

Myotomy, tenotomy, (controlled or bridled) advancement or shortening of ocular muscles; Tenon's capsule incision.

Muscle transplantation.

Orbit

Incision

Orbitotomy (anterior or lateral): Opening of the orbit for removal of cysts, neoplasms and foreign bodies.

Introduction

Orbital injection of alcohol for hemorrhagic glaucoma or intractable pain.

Cautery puncture: To induce slight cicatricial contraction in the orbicularis muscle and make adhesions between it and the tarsus.

Repair

Plastic repair of orbit.

Orbicularis resection.

Eyelids

Incision

Canthotomy: Slitting of the canthus.

Tarsotomy: Incision of tarsal cartilage of an eyelid.

Blepharotomy: Incision of an eyelid.

Tarsectomy: Surgical removal of tarsal plate of an eyelid.

Recession of levator palpebrae muscle.

Excision

Blepharectomy: Incision or excision of

meibomian cyst, tumor of a meibomian gland.

Tarsectomy: Excision of a segment of the tarsus of an eyelid.

Repair

Blepharoplasty: Surgical restoration of eyelid and eyebrow.

Canthoplasty: Division to lengthen the upper lid at the lateral canthus.

Plastic restoration of eyebrow (by graft).

Electrolysis: For the inversion of a few distorted cilia at either one or several sites on the lid margin.

Tarsoplasty, Blepharoplasty: Plastic surgery of margin or eyelid.

Reposition of ciliary base.

Tarsal paring and eversion: To prevent corneal ulceration.

Tarsocheiloplasty: Plastic surgery of borders of the eyelid.

Tarsal Rotation operation: Fashioning of a new intermarginal strip to correct entropin of the upper lid in the late stage of trachoma.

Suture

Blepharorrhaphy: Suture of eyelid.

Tarsorrhaphy: Surgical uniting of the edges of the lids at the outer commissure to reduce width of palpebral fissure, or to protect cornea.

Canthorrhaphy: Suture of eyelids at either canthus.

Conjunctiva

Incision

Removal of foreign body from surface of conjunctiva.

Suture of conjunctiva.

Excision

Biopsy of conjunctiva.

Excision of lesion of conjunctiva.

Repair

Conjunctivoplasty: Surgical removal of part of cornea, but replacing with flaps from conjunctiva.

Flap operation for corneal ulcer.

Flap operation: "Flapping" of conjunctiva for perforating injuries of operative wound for laceration.

Lacrimal Tract

Incision

Lacrimotomy: Surgical incision of the lacrimal duct.

Dacrocystostomy: Incision of the lacrimal sac with drainage.

Dacrocystosyringotomy: Incising the lacrimal sac and duct.

Dacrocystotomy: Surgical incision of the tear sac.

Excision

Dacrocystectomy: Excision of the wall of the lacrimal sac.

Dacroadenectomy: Excision of a lacrimal gland.

Dacrocystectomy: Excision of the wall of the lacrimal sac.

Repair

Dacryocystorhinostomy: Surgical formation of a communication between the lacrimal sac and the middle meatus of the nose through the lacrimal bone.

Dacryorhinocystotomy: An operation of passing a probe through the lacrimal sac and into the nasal cavity.

Filtration Operations

These procedures are performed to (1) effect permanent channels for the seepage of aqueous from the anterior chamber to the subconjunctival tissue; (2) To effect a filtering cicatrix along the track of a piece of iris included in a scleral incision; (3) Goniotomy: To open the filtration angle by stripping and peeling from the posterior surface of the cornea, the iris and congenital mesoplastic tissue at this site; and (4) Trephine operations: To effect a filtering cicatrix over the filtration angle through which aqueous may seep and drain away beneath the conjunctiva, thus decompressing the eye.

Evisceration

Removal of the contents of the eyeball.

Evisceroneurotomy: Scleral evisceration of the eye with division of the optic nerve.

Air Injection

Intra-ocular injection of air in eye surgery is used in the field of anatomical restoration and replacement.

In cyclodialyses operations air injected into the anterior chamber, widens and keeps open the intra-ocular filtration track between the filtration angle and the suprachoroidal lymph space; and again, reforms the anterior chamber.

NOSE

The nose is the peripheral organ of smell, and it consists of the external nose and the nasal cavities with the essential olfactory mucous membrane. Respiration and olfaction (smell) are the two major functions of the nose (Plate 39). By warming, moistening and filtering the inspired air, the nose prepares the air for use in the respiratory passages. In addition, the other important functions are associated with phonation (resonating chamber), ventilation and drainage. Hypo- or hyperfunctional responses may be caused by physical, constitutional, febrile, emotional, allergic and environmental states.

The following factors are essential for normal function of the nose:
1. Large surface area (turbinates).
2. Moist surface (mucous sheath).
3. Movement and replenishment of sheath (celia and glands).
4. Heat supply (cavernous spaces).
5. Proper biochemical composition (pH) of nasal secretion.
6. Normal pathway for air.

The external nose has the shape of an irregular triangular pyramid and is connected on its base surface (basio nasi) with the skeleton of the face and at its margin projects from the region of the upper jaw. The upper narrow end joining the forehead is called the radix nasi (the root of the nose), and from this the dorsum nasi (back of the nose) passes downward obliquely and forward to the tip of the nose (the apex nasi). The lateral surfaces of the nose are curved below, project more and are limited laterally by a sharp groove, which restricts this movable part, nasal wings (alae nasi). Its lower free margin (margo nasi) surrounds the nasal openings, the anterior nares. The latter are separated by the most anterior movable part of the nasal septum, septum mobile nasi (columnella). Thus, the nose has a heart-shaped base with two symmetrical elliptical nostrils.

The external nasal framework is formed by the nasal bones and hyaline cartilages. Muscle and skin cover the external surface of these structures; the inner surface is lined with mucous membrane except for a small anterior area, vestibuli nasi, which is covered by skin continuous with that of the face.

The nasal septum constitutes a medial wall of each nasal cavity, consisting of one particularly large cartilaginous and four osseous plates, all firmly united to divide the nasal cavity into two chambers.

The osseous nasal cavity is divided into a right and left cavity (cavum nasi) (anterior nares) to the environment; posteriorly (choanae) to the nasopharyngeal space.

The process of filtering inspired air is an important function. The vibrissae within the vestibules of the nares filters out coarse particles. The filtering of dust and bacteria on the mucous membrane is further facilitated by the adhesive property of the mucous; thus the filtered substance deposited in the mucous membrane is disposed of through the action of the cilia.

The specilized sense of smell receives its stimuli from olfactory receptors in the olfactory portion of the nasal mucous membrane. To produce this stimuli, substances must be finely divided and conveyed by an upward direction of air in the nasal chamber.

SURGICAL PROCEDURES—NOSE

Nose

Incision
  Drainage of nasal abscess.
  Drainage of septal abscess.

Excision
  Biopsy, soft tissue, nose.
  Excision of nasal polyp.
  Excision of nasal polyps, multiple (unilateral or bilateral).
  Intranasal excision of kyphosis or hump.
  Excision of skin of nose for rhinophyma—enlargement and redness of the entire nose with large blood vessels in the skin of nose.

Repair
  Rhinokyphectomy: A rhinoplastic operation for kyphosis by intranasal excision of the hump.
  Rhinopolasty: Surgical formation of a new nose.

Rhinochiloplasty: Plastic surgery of the nose and lip.

Destruction

Cauterization of turbinates, unilateral or bilateral.

Manipulation

Reduction of fractured nasal bones.

Control of primary nasal hemorrhage, with cauterization of septum, or with nasal pack. By ligation of ethmoid artery.

TONGUE

The tongue (lingua) is a movable muscular organ on the floor of the mouth, subserving the special sense of taste and aiding in mastication, deglutition and articulation of sound. It ends in front in a flat, rounded tip (*apex linguae*). Following upon this is the body of the tongue, the *corpus linguae*, which is in turn bounded behind by the *sulcus terminalis*, the right and left limbs of which run obliquely backward toward the median plane and meet in the *foramen caecum linguae (Morgagnii)*. The area behind the *sulcus terminalis* is called the *radix linguae* (root of the tongue). The upper surface of the tongue (*dorsum linguae*) is curved in a sagittal and frontal direction so as to be convex upward and presents in the median plane in front a shallow groove, the *sulcus medianus (linguae)*. The body of the tongue is bounded laterally by the *Margo lateralis (linguae)*. The inferior surface, *facies inferior (linguae)*, lies free only along its lateral margins and below the anterior portion of the tongue.

The tongue is covered with mucous membrane and the upper surface is studded with *papillae*. The *papillae* give the tongue its rough appearance and of these *papillae*, there are four varieties: (1) vallate, or circumvallate, papillae which are near the root of the tongue and contain the taste buds; (2) fungiform papillae, which resemble fungi in shape and are found on the tip and sides of the tongue; (3) filiform papillae cover the interior two-thirds of the tongue, bear delicate brushlike processes, seem to be connected with the sense of touch and are very highly developed on the tip of the tongue; (4) simple papillae like those of the skin cover the larger papillae and all of the mucous membrane of the dorsum of the tongue.

TASTE BUDS

The many wonderful flavors we distinguish are the products of sweet, sour, salt and bitter basic tastes. And, still more remarkable is the fact that this minute differentiation of so many flavors depends upon the tiny bud-shaped bodies, the *taste buds*. The taste buds are most numerous upon the mucous membrane of the tongue, particularly in the walls of the moats surrounding the vallate papillae, but also sparsely found on the oral surface of the soft palate and on the posterior aspect of the epiglottis. Taste buds consist of supporting cells shaped like slices of melon surrounded by several layers like the staves of a barrel, the special neuroepithelial or gustatory cells, which leave at the apex of the bud a small pit which communicates with the surface by a fine gustatory pore. Scattered among the supporting cells in the center of the bud are the long narrow epithelial taste cells, their free ends extending to the pit into which each sends a short, fine gustatory hair. Terminal fibers from the nerves of taste enter the deep end of the taste bud to send fibrils between gustatory cells. Substances to be tasted after dissolving in saliva and reaching the pit by the pore so stimulate the hairs of the neuroepithelial cells that impulses are conveyed in their associated nerve fibers to the brain for analysis.

Nerves of Taste

The chorda tympani nerve transmits taste fibers from the anterior two-thirds of the tongue. Nerve fibers terminating in the tongue are fibers of: (1) the lingual nerve, a sensory branch of the fifth or trigeminal; (2) the chorda tympani, a branch of the seventh or facial nerve, which transmits taste fibers from the anterior two-thirds of the tongue; (3) the ninth or glossopharyngeal nerve; and (4) the twelfth or hypoglossal nerve is a motor nerve distributed to the tongue.

The glossopharyngeal nerve transmits taste fibers from the posterior third, vallate papillae and soft palate, the greater superficial petrosal, also from the soft palate and the internal laryngeal from the posterior surface of the epiglottis. The taste fibers in these nerves are the peripheral processes of unipolar nerve cells in the ganglia of the facial, glossopharyngeal and vagus nerves, while the central processes end in the nucleus of the tractus solitarius.

IV

DISEASES

Disease is a definite morbid process having a characteristic train of symptoms, which may effect the whole body or any of its parts, and its etiology, pathology, and prognosis may be known or unknown.

A disease is a pathological condition of the body that presents a group of symptoms peculiar to it, and which sets the condition apart as an abnormal entity differing from other normal or pathological body states.

Topography: Classification of the location of a disease.

Etiology: Study of the cause of disease which results in pathological conditions.

Pathology: That branch of medicine which treats of the essential nature of the disease, especially of the structural and functional changes in tissues and organs of the body which cause or are caused by disease.

Prognosis: A forecast as to the probable result of an attack of disease; the prospect as to recovery from a disease as indicated by the nature and symptoms of the case.

Disease Conditions

Acute: Having a rapid onset.

Chronic: Having a slow onset and having lasted for a long period of time.

Communicable: The infection in nature of which is transmissible from one person to another; either directly or indirectly through a carrier or vector.

Congenital: A disease which is present at birth and may be due to hereditary factors or prenatal infection.

Constitutional: A disease which is due to an individual's hereditary make-up involving the body as a whole in contrast to one involving specific organs.

Contagious: An infectious disease readily transmitted from one person to another, usually within a short period of time.

Deficiency: A disease resulting from inadequate intake or absorption of essential dietary factors such as vitamins or minerals.

Degenerative: A disease resulting from degenerative changes that occur in tissues and organs, characteristic of old age.

Endemic: A disease which is present more or less continuously in a community.

Epidemic: A disease which attacks a large number of individuals in a community at the same time.

Familial: A disease which occurs in several individuals of the same family.

Functional: A disease in which no anatomical changes can be observed to account for the symptoms present.

Hereditary: A disease due to hereditary factors transmitted from parent to offspring.

Iatrogenic: A disease resulting from the activity of physicians, e.g., a term applied to disorders induced in the patient by autosuggestion based on the physician's examination, manner or discussion, (Sir Arthur Hurst).

Idiopathic: A disease for which no causative factor can be recognized.

Infectious: A disease resulting from the presence in the body of a pathogenic organism.

Malignant: A disease in which the progress is extremely rapid, generally threatening or resulting in death within a short time.

Occupational: A disease resulting from factors associated with the occupation engaged in by the individual.

Organic: A disease resulting from factors recognizable as anatomic changes in an organ, or tissue of the body.

Pandemic: An epidemic disease which is extremely widespread involving an entire country, continent or possibly the entire world.

Parasitic: A disease resulting from the growth and development of parasitic organisms (plant or animals) in, or upon the body.

Periodic: A disease that occurs at more-or-less regular intervals or at the same time each year.

Psychosomatic: A disease in which structural changes in or malfunctioning of organs are due to the mind, especially the emotions.

Sporadic: A disease in which only occasional cases occur; not epidemic or endemic.

Subacute: A disease in which symptoms are less pronounced, but more prolonged than in an acute disease; intermediate between acute and chronic disease.

Venereal: V.D. (abbreviation) includes syphilis, gonorrhea and chancroid, and is usually acquired through sexual relations.

V

ANESTHESIOLOGY

Anesthesiology is the science of anesthesia. Anesthesia is a partial or complete loss of sensation, with or without loss of consciousness, as a result of disease, injury or administration of a drug or gas.

TYPES OF ANESTHESIA

Block   Resulting from nerve blocking by injection of alcohol or other substance, into or very near to a nerve trunk.

Bulbar   Pons lesion causing central anesthesia.

Caudal   Spinal anesthesia induced by injection in region of cauda (equina), or sacral canal.

Controlled Dolitrone: It is injected into the veins and although the patient has no sense of pain he can talk and obey orders but will not remember any of his experience while under the drug.

Dolorsa   Painfulness of a part with anesthesia of that part, as in thalmic lesions.

General   One that is complete and affecting the entire body with loss of consciousness, when the anesthetic acts upon the brain.

Infiltration   Local anesthesia achieved by injecting a weak coccaine solution.

Inhalation   General anesthesia achieved by inhaling ether or chloroform vapors or nitrous oxide gas.

Local   One effecting a local area only, the anesthetic upon nerves or nerve tracts.

Mixed   Producing a general anesthesia by more than one drug, as nitrous gas, continued by ether.

Neural   Injection of an anesthetic into a nerve or immediately around it (intraneural and paraneural).

Primary   First stage of anesthesia.

Rectal   General anesthesia produced by introduction of an anesthetic agent into rectum.

Regional   Nerve or field blocking, causing insensibility over a particular area.

Spinal or Spinal puncture   When the injection into the theca is up to a level at which nerves of the area enter the spinal cord.

Surgical   When depth of anesthesia produces relaxation of muscles and loss of sensation or consciousness.

Twilight   State of light anesthesia induced to alleviate labor pains.

ANESTHETIC AGENTS

General	Local
Oxygen (O_2)	Chlorprocaine (Nescaine)
Hydrogen (H_2)	Cocaine Hydrochloride (cocaine)
Ether	Cyclomethycaine (Surfacaine)
Chloroform	Dibucaine (suppositories) (Nupercaine)
Ethyl—vinyl e. (Vinethene)	Ethyl chloride
Ethyl chloride	Lidocaine HCL (Xylocaine)
Nitrous oxide	Lidocaine HCL with epinephrine
Ethylene	Piperocaine HCL
Helium (He)	Procaine HCL
Cyclopropane	Tetracaine HCL
Acetylene	Metycaine HCL
Halothane (Fluothane)	
Tribromoethanol	Procain
Dimethyl e.	Novocain
Penthrane (methoxyflurane)	Pontocaine
	Nupercaine
	Surfacaine
	Xylocaine

100

Inhalation	Intravenous	Basal post-operative	Block, Regional, Spinal
Fluothane	Brevital sodium	Amytal	Blockaine, hydro-chloride
Halothane	Pentothal		
2-Bromo-chloro-1	Surital	Noctec	Carbocaine
		Pentothal sodium	Cyclaine
1-Trifluoroethane	Viadril	Seconal	Nesacaine
Vinethene		Tuinal	Sarapin
Vinyl ether		Viadril	Xylocaine
Pure vinyl ether			

Local, Eye	Muscular	Relaxants
Enzodase	Tubarine	d-Tubo-chloride
Vanlint	curarine	
Wydase		

VI

RADIOLOGY

Radiology is that branch of medicine dealing with X-rays and radioactive materials and generally divided into three groups: diagnostic radiology, therapeutic radiology and nuclear medicine.

Diagnostic radiology is concerned with the diagnosis of disease by means of pictures produced by passing X-rays through the body. It is common practice to enhance contrast by using a radiopaque material to cast a dense shadow, as barium in studies of the gastrointestinal tract and iodinated compounds when studying the vascular system and urinary tract.

Therapeutic radiology deals mainly with the treatment of cancer by passing carefully directed and sized beams through the area of the tumor or diseased area. The energy used in therapeutic radiology usually runs 10 to 20 times higher or more than that used in diagnostic radiology.

Nuclear medicine deals with the diagnosis and treatment by means of radioactive isotopes. The most widely known and used is radioactive iodine (^{131}I) in the diagnosis and treatment of thyroid disease.

Cinefluorography is the use of a permanent photographic recording by motion picture camera of a fluoroscopic X-ray image.

Fluoroscopy is a technique for producing a temporary image of objects interposed between the X-ray source, and a screen coated with calcium tungstate or other fluorescing crystals.

GENERAL PROPERTIES OF ROENTGEN RAYS

The usefulness of roentgen rays in the practice of medicine depends on several general properties. In diagnosis these are:

1. The ability of roentgen rays to penetrate some objects and substances opaque to ordinary light.

2. The ability of roentgen rays to affect a photographic emulsion.

3. The ability of roentgen rays to cause fluorescence of certain crystals.

In addition, roentgen rays have very important biological effects upon which their usefulness in therapy depends. They also possess the power of ionizing gases, a property used in accurate measurements of intensities of exposure to treatments.

PENETRATING POWER OF ROENTGEN RAYS

The penetrability of a substance by roentgen rays depends on the nature of the substance, its thickness and the quality of the rays attempting to pass through it. Thus, rays just penetrating enough to pass through a thin part such as the hand would all be absorbed by a thicker part, such as the hip.

The penetrating power of roentgen rays depends on their wave-lengths—the shorter the rays, the greater the penetrability. Since the wave lengths are determined by the voltage of the current producing the rays, penetrability may be determined and expressed in terms of voltage. This makes it possible, without making an actual determination of the wave-lengths to indicate a certain quality of rays, both in wavelengths and in penetrability, by mentioning the voltage at which they were produced; a rough measure of quality, which is the common and usual practice in roentgenography.

EFFECT OF ROENTGEN RAYS ON PHOTOGRAPHIC EMULSION

An important property of roentgen rays is their ability to affect a photographic emulsion in a manner similar to visible light. A photographic emulsion is made of a preparation of silver bromide suspended in an emulsion of gelatin and spread in a thin layer on some form of support; if on a transparent, celluloid-like base, a film is the result. The base of a double-coated X-ray film is made of cellulose acetate of sufficient thickness to provide a certain amount of rigidity. Usually a small amount of bluish dye is incorporated in the base, to give more of a white light when films are examined, thus in a measure offsetting the yellowish light of a viewing apparatus. Two kinds of films with different emulsions are currently produced for general roentgenographic work. On screen-exposure films, the emulsion is made particularly sensitive to the bluish and ultraviolet radiation from intensifying screens.

PROCESSING OF X-RAY FILMS

It is said that a "latent image" is formed in the emulsion. When an X-ray film is exposed, a change takes place in the silver halides in the emulsion wherein small amounts of impurity, usually sulfur, in the silver bromide crystal form small "trapping centers" of silver sulfide for electrons within the normal lattice of the crystal. By a series of electron transfer, a silver ion eventually combines with an electron (both products of exposure to ionizing radiation) to form metallic silver, which then acts as the nucleus for deposition of the remaining silver of the individual crystal during processing.

When an exposed film is placed in a solution known as a developing solution or developer, the chemicals change the silver of the latent image to metallic granules or particles (known as a reducing action) held in place by the gelatin of the emulsion. The silver that is not affected by the X-ray exposure remains unchanged. It is removed by placing the film in a second solution known as a fixing bath. In this the unaffected silver is dissolved from the film. Washing of the films to remove the fixing-bath chemicals and drying them to remove the water complete the processing.

ROENTGENOGRAMS

When a roentgenogram is examined with a suitable viewing light, it is seen to be made up of lighter and darker portions. The lighter and darker areas on roentgenograms represent the differences in the density of the structures or parts of the body through which the rays have passed to reach the intensifying screens. Thus, the film, the finished roentgenogram, is a shadowgraphic pictoral representation of these differences in density. When structures of considerable difference in density such as bone and flesh lie side by side, their differentiation is marked; if the differences in density are slight, as between the kidneys and the surrounding tissues, the shadows will show but little variation in shade. If there is no appreciable difference in density of the two structures lying side by side, neither will be lighter nor darker than the other, and there will be no differentiation on the film. On soft tissue roentgenograms, the shadows of muscle masses, facial planes, tendons and even some blood vessels may be dense enough to be pictured as lighter shades of gray than surrounding subcutaneous fat. Air in the lungs, in the nasal accessory sinuses and in the mastoid cells, and air or gas in the alimentary canal decreases density and causes darker shadows than surrounding structures—bone on the other hand is white on roetgenograms.

ROENTGENOGRAPHIC PROCEDURES

Chest
Bedside
Bronchography, with or without injection
Fluoroscopy
Laminography
Ribs, sternum
Routine (Stereo, PA lateral)
Sinus tract study (with injection)
Special (grid, oblique lordotic)

Gastrointestinal Tract
Acute abdomen series
Cholangiography (I.V.), or with injection
Colon (all types)
Esophagus special
Fluoroscopy (Tube passage)
Gall Bladder (Cholecystography)
Sinus tract study (with injection)

Small bowel special
Upper gastrointestinal (GI series)

Spine
Cervical
Discography
Dorsal
Sinogram—sinus tract study, usually with injection of radiopaque material
Laminography
Lumbosacral
Myelography
Sacroiliac
Scoliotic
Special (obliques)

Lower Extremity
Ankle
Arthrogram (with injection of air or radiopaque material)
Femur
Foot, toes
Hip nailing series
Hip (AP lateral)
Knee
Laminography
Pelvis (AP only)
Teleroentgenography
Tibia, fibula

Upper Extremity
Clavicle
Elbow
Hand, fingers
Humerus
Laminography
Radius, ulna
Shoulder, scapula
Skeletal survey
Wrist
Bone age survey

Skull, Brain
Arteriography, carotid or vertebral
Encephalogram
Pneumoencephalogram (without injection)
Laminography
Routine skull
Special
Stereotaxic study
Ventriculogram, air (without injection), or opaque (without injection)

Head, Neck
Facial bones
Laminography
Mandible
Mastoids
Neck, soft tissues
Ocular foreign body localization
Sialography (without injection)
Sinuses
Temporomandibular Joints

Urinary Tract
Cystography
KUB survey film
Nephrography (with injection)
Pneumography (without injection)
Urethrocystography (with injection)
Urography, excretory (with injection)
Urography, retrograde

Female Reproductive System
Hysterosalpingo (without injection)
Obstetrical routine
Pelvimetry special
Placental localization

Cardiovascular System
Angio-selective (without catheterization)
Angio-venous (without injection)
Aortography-abdomen (without injection)
Aortography-thoracic (without catheterization)
Arteriography-periphers (without injection)
Arteriography-visceral (without catheterization)
Heart film series
Heart fluoroscopy
Kymography
Venography-peripheral (without injection)
Venography-portal (without injection)

Radiation Therapy

Cancer of Cervix
1. Intrauterine radium
2. Vaginal radium
3. Special radium
4. Pelvic irradiation
5. Transvaginal

Cancer of Corpus Uteri
1. Vaginal radium
2. Intrauterine radium
3. Pelvic irradiation

Cancer of Ovary
1. Pelvic irradiation
2. Abdominal irradiation

Cancer of Vagina or Vulva
1. Interstitial radium
2. Applicator radium
3. External irradiation

Radiation Castration
1. Short
2. Protracted

Cancer of Testis
1. Pelvic and abdominal irradiation
2. Irradiation of mediastinum

Cancer of Bladder
1. External irradiation
2. Central source isotope
3. Interstitial implant

Cancer of Kidney
1. External irradiation

Cancer of Liver
1. External irradiation

Cancer of Pancreas
1. External irradiation

Cancer of Nasal Fossa
1. External irradiation

Cancer of Nasopharynx
1. External irradiation

Cancer of Sinuses
1. External irradiation
2. Intercavitary radium

Cancer of Pharynx, Hypopharynx, Piriform Fossa
1. External irradiation

Cancer of Larynx
1. External irradiation

Cancer of Bronchus
1. Mediastinal irradiation
2. External irradiation of primary lesion

Cancer of Pleura
1. External irradiation
2. Isotope irradiation

Cancer of Skin
1. Face
2. Eyelid
3. Pinna
4. Trunk, Extremities

Hemangioma
1. External irradiation

Brain Tumor
1. External irradiation

Pituitary Adenoma

Cancer of Conjunctiva
1. External irradiation
2. Applicator

Pterygium
1. Applicator

Retinoblastoma
1. External irradiation

Retrobulbar Lymphoma
1. External irradiation

Malignant Exophthalmus
1. External irradiation

Neuroblastoma

Bone Tumors
1. Giant cell tumor
2. Ewing's
3. Multiple myeloma
4. Xanthomatosis
5. Metastatic

Soft Tissue and Retroperitoneal Tumors

Hodgkins Disease
1. Mediastinum
2. Sterilization of nodes
3. Palliation, nodes

Lymphosarcoma

Chronic Leukemia

Irradiation of Nodes or Spleen

Bursitis

Cellulitis

Parotitis

Recurrent Otitis Media
1. Pharyngeal irradiation

Peptic Ulcer, Gastric Suppression

Herpes Zoster

Rheumatoid Spondylitis

Hyperthyroidism, Treatment ^{131}I

Carcinoma of Thyroid ^{131}I

Treatment of Malignant Effusions
1. Radioactive chronic phosphate
2. ^{198}Au

Wilms Tumor
1. Abdominal and Pelvic irradiation

Cancer of Urethra
1. External irradiation

Cancer of Prostate
1. External irradiation
2. Interstitial irradiation

Cancer of Breast
1. Routine postoperative
2. Chest wall external irradiation
3. Chest wall implant
4. Metastases
   a. Single site
   b. Multiple sites

Cancer of Lip
1. Routine or complicated

Cancer Buccal Mucosa
1. External irradiation
2. Radium mould

Cancer Alveolar Ridge
1. External irradiation

Cancer of Palate
1. External irradiation

Cancer, Floor of Mouth
1. External irradiation
2. Radium mould
3. Interstitial implant

Cancer, Anterior Tongue
1. External irradiation
2. Interstitial irradiation

Cancer, Base of Tongue
1. External irradiation
2. Interstitial irradiation

Cancer, Tonsil
1. External irradiation

Cancer, Salivary Glands
1. External irradiation
2. Interstitial implant

Metastatic Nodes in Neck (Inoperable)
1. External irradiation
2. Interstitial implant

Cancer of Esophagus
1. External irradiation

Cancer of Anus
1. External irradiation

Cancer of Anus
1. External irradiation
2. Interstitial irradiation

Cancer of Colon
1. External irradiation

VII

PATHOLOGY

Pathology is that branch of medicine which treats of the essential nature of the disease, especially of the structural and functional changes in tissues and organs of the body which cause or are caused by disease.

KINDS OF PATHOLOGICAL CONDITIONS

Cellular: That which regards the cells as starting points of the phenomena of disease and that every cell descends from some pre-existing cell (Virchow).

Clinical: Pathology applied to the solution of clinical problems; especially the use of laboratory methods in clinical diagnosis.

Comparative: That which constitutes comparisons between various diseases of the human body and those of the lower animals.

Dental: The sum of knowledge regarding diseases of the teeth.

Exotic: A system of pathology foreign to the country or school in which it has found a lodgment.

Experimental: The study of artificially induced disease processes.

Functional: The study of changes of function due to morbid tissue changes.

General: That which takes cognizance of pathologic conditions which may occur in various diseases and in different organs.

Geographical: Pathology in its geographic and climatic relations.

Humoral: The opinion that disease is due to abnormal conditions of the fluids of the body.

Internal: Medical pathology.

Medical: That which relates to morbid processes which are not accessible to operative intervention.

Mental: Psychopathology.

Plant: Vegetable pathology.

Solidistic: That opinion which attributes disease to rarefaction or condensation of the solid tissues.

PATHOLOGICAL EXAMINATIONS

Blood
Agglutinations for febrile diseases
Alcohol, blood
Amylase, blood
Antistreptolysin titer
Ascorbic acid
Basophilic aggregates (L-E cells)
Bilirubin (Van den Bergh)
Bleeding time
Blood culture, aerobic and anaerobic
Blood, red cell count
    hemoglobin determination, photoelectric
    white cell count
    differential count
    complete blood count
Bone marrow, collection and examination of material
Bromides
Bromosulphalein
C-reactive protein
Calcium
Carbon dioxide combining power
Congo red
Cephalin flocculation
Arterial puncture
CO_2 content arterial blood
Chlorides

Cholesterol
Cholesterol ester
Clot reaction
Coagulation time (Lee & White) or other methods
Complement fixation tests (Wassermann, etc.)
Complement fixation, quantitative
Treponema pallidum immobilization
Creatinine
Creatinine clearance
Creatine
Electrophoresis pattern, protein, lipoprotein
Eosinophil count
Flocculation tests (Kline, Kahn, etc.)
Hemoglobin, carbon monoxide
    methemoglobin
    sulfhemoglobin
Hematocrit
Heterophile antibody with absorption, or without
Oxygen saturation, arterial blood
pH (arterial or venous blood)
Icterus index
Lead
Lipase
Lipids, total
Phospholipids
Non-protein nitrogen
O_2 Content (arterial blood)
Blood oxygen
Oxycorticoids
Phosphatase, acid, or alkaline
Phosphorus
Platelet count
Potassium
Protein bound iodine
Prothrombin time
Prothrombin utilization
Red cell fragility
Reticulocyte count
Rh titer
Sedimentation rate
Smears for parasites (malaria, etc.)
Sodium
Sugar
Sugar tolerance, 3 hours, 5 hours
Sulfonamide blood level
Thymol turbidity
Total protein
    and albumin/globulin ration
Albumin/globulin ratio

Typing blood
Rh
Coombs technique
Crossmatch, saline and albumin
Urea
Urea clearance
Uric acid
Vitamin A
Volume, blood (dye method)
Radioisotopes

Feces
Occult blood
Routine chemical, fat, starch
Routine microscopic, wet preparation (parasites)
Iron hematoxylin stain
Routine chemical and microscopic examination, including parasites
Routine to include complete chemical and microscopic (series of three)
Quantitative urobilinogen
Culture for bacteria, screening, definitive

Gastric or Duodenal Contents (Includes Aspiration)
Gastric contents, sterile technique, microscopic, chemical acid, fractional, with histamine, augmented histamine, chemical, pepsin tubeless
Duodenal contents, microscopic enzyme determination as ordered
Smear for TB, concentrated
Culture for TB, concentrated

Spinal Fluid
Spinal fluid collection
Routine chemical (Pandy)
Routine microscopic (cell count)
Routine chemical and microscopic
Colloidal gold (mastic, carbon, etc.)
Complement fixation tests for syphilis
Smear for bacteria
Culture for bacteria screening, definitive
Quantitative chemical tests (as per blood)

Sputum
Smear, direct; after concentration
Gastric or tracheal wash with culture for tubercle bacilli

Culture, direct, screening, direct definitive
 after concentration,
 for fungus

Tissues

Surgical, gross only
 gross and microscopic
 frozen section (includes permanent section)
 culture for bacteria screening; definitive
Cytologic study (Papanicolaou smear)
 gastric or pepsin

Urine

Urinary determination of free gastric acidity by colorimetric dye study
Routine chemical, qualitative
 qualitative, sugar
Routine microscopic
Bence-Jones protein
Complete routine (chemical and microscopic)
Quantitative functional (Addis)
Concentration and dilution tests
Sugar fermentation
Phenosulfonphthalein
Porphyrins, qualitative, quantitative
Smear for bacteria
Porphobilinogen
Culture for bacteria screening
Lead, quantitative
Culture for bacteria, definitive
Quantitative calcium (Sulkowitch)
Bile pigments
Quantitative chemical examination
24 hour calcium

Miscellaneous

Antibiotic sensitivity, per antibiotic (pyrogenic)

Antibiotic sensitivity (Tbc.)
Audiometer testing, any method
Barany vestibular test
Basal metabolic rate
Electrocardiogram with interpretation and report
Biologic test for pregnancy (A-Z, Friedman, etc.)
 Frog
Darkfield examinations skin lesion, blood
Urinary hormone determinations:
 (a) 17-ketosteroids
 (b) 11-oxysteroids
 (c) Gonadotropins
 (d) Pregnanediol
Residual air determination
Exclusion test for pheochromoctoma (Regitine, etc .)
Direct smear without stain
Miscellaneous smear for bacteria with stain
Miscellaneous culture for bacteria screening
Guinea pig for Tbc
Miscellaneous animal inoculation for bacteria
Miscellaneous culture for bacteria definitive
Vital capacity
Skin tests with bacterial extracts (Brucella, Frei, Tuberculin, etc.)
Venous pressure
Circulation time
Stone analysis, qualitative
 quantitative
Transudates and exudates, microscopic
Culture screening
 definitive
Animal inoculation

BIBLIOGRAPHY

1. *Dorland's Illustrated Medical Dictionary*, ed. 23. W. B. Saunders Co., Philadelphia, 1958.
2. *Dorland's Illustrated Medical Dictionary*, ed. 24. W. B. Saunders Co., Philadelphia, 1965.
3. Gray, H.: *Anatomy of the Human Body*, edited by W. H. Lewis, ed. 24. Lea and Febiger, Philadelphia, 1942.
4. Gray, H.: *Anatomy of the Human Body*, edited by C. M. Goss, ed. 27. Lea and Febiger, Philadelphia, 1959.
5. Kimber, D. C., and Gray, C. E.: *Textbook of Anatomy and Physiology*, edited by C. E. Stackpole and L. C. Leavell, ed. 13. The MacMillan Co., New York, 1957.
6. King, B. G., and Showers, M. J.: *Human Anatomy and Physiology*, ed. 5. W. B. Saunders Co., Philadelphia, 1963.
7. Lederer, F. L., and Hollender, A. R.: *Basic Otolaryngology*, ed. 4. F. A. Davis Co., Philadelphia, 1956.
8. Lockhart, R. D., Hamilton, G. F., and Fyee, F. W.: *Anatomy of the Human Body*. J. B. Lippincott Co., Philadelphia, 1959.
9. Millard, N. D., King, B. G., and Showers, M. J.: *Human Anatomy and Physiology*, ed. 4. W. B. Saunders Co., Philadelphia, 1956.
10. Montagna, W.: *The Structure and Function of Skin*, ed. 2. Academic Press, Inc., New York, 1962.
11. Ranson, S. W.: *The Anatomy of the Nervous System. Its Development and Function*, revised by S. L. Clark, ed. 9. W. B. Saunders Co., Philadelphia, 1953.
12. Rhinehart, D. A.: *Roentgenographic Technique*, ed. 4. Lea and Febiger, Philadelphia, 1954.
13. *Stedman's Medical Dictionary*, ed. 20. The Williams & Wilkins Co., Baltimore, 1961.
14. *Taber's Cyclopedic Medical Dictionary*, ed. 8. F. A. Davis Co., Philadelphia, 1958.
15. Woodbine, R. T.: *Essentials of Human Anatomy*, ed. 2. Oxford University Press, New York, 1961.